Calorie, Fat & Carbohydrate Counter

Calorie, Fat & Carbohydrate Counter

Compiled by Anne Fennell

Capella

First published in Great Britain by
Arcturus Publishing Limited
1–7 Shand Street
London SE1 2ES

For Bookmart Limited
Registered Number 2372865
Desford Road
Enderby
Leicester LE19 4AD

This edition published 2002.

Cover design by Alex Ingr
Text design by Viki Ottewill

Printed and bound by
Nørhaven Paperback A/S, Viborg

ISBN 1-84193-144-6

Contents

2 DRINKS

3 BREAKFAST FOODS

4 LUNCHTIME FOODS

5 COOKED MEALS

6 SWEETS AND DESSERTS

7 FAST FOOD

8 ALPHABETICAL LISTING OF MOST COMMON FOODS

Introduction

Our body is the most wonderful machine. Like a car needs fuel to keep it running, our body needs food to be able to carry out its daily needs. To reach its maximum potential the body needs the right amount of food; too much and one feels bloated and lethargic; too little and one feels weak and ill. As one dietician instructed: "Half fill the stomach with food and a quarter with liquid, leaving a quarter empty so that the digesting process can work properly. If one fills the stomach with food, one must use extra energy, acids and liquids to digest it, and then, at the next time, the supplied energy, acids and liquids will be short and trouble will start. The undigested food creates different types of liquids and acids which destroy the blood and result in skin diseases, obesity and sickness. If, on the other hand, one takes too little food, then the body machine will start eating itself, and again loss of energy is the result."

This is a direction that can be followed by anyone. As a rule half the energy provided by food is used to maintain the bodily functions, the other half is used by activities such as work, play, sport etc. If one eats more food than is needed the excess will be stored by the body as fat and the body will put on weight. On the whole active people use more energy and will need to eat more to meet their energy requirements.

Energy provided by food and used by the body is measured in calories (kcal). The rate at which the body uses up calories varies according to age, weight, sex, and fitness. For an average female, weighing about 9 stone (57kg), aged between 18-35yrs old, leading a reasonably active life the daily calories needed is roughly 2,100. For an average man following the same description, weighing about 12 stone (75kg) 3,150 calories are required daily. For a woman, weighing 9 stone (57kg), aged between 35-55yrs old, leading a reasonably active life, 1,900 calories are needed. For a man, following the same description, weighing about 12 stone (75kg), 2,800 calories are required. For a woman over 55 years, weighing 9 stone (57kg), 1,600 calories are required. For a man over 55 years, weighing about 12 stone (75kg), 2,400 calories are required. Please note these are only rough guidelines for an average person leading a moderately active life. Individual requirements vary.

Carbohydrates

Carbohydrates are a major source of energy in the diet and should make up half of the calories we eat. Carbohydrates are divided into two main types: starches, consisting of bread, rice, pasta and potatoes and sugars. Sugars are of three different types: sugars not found within the cellular structure of food such as confectionery, biscuits, table sugar, soft drinks, cakes etc; sugars that are found in vegetables and fruit; and sugars that are found in milk and its products. As is well known it is the sugars of the first type, that tend to be over-indulged, that lead to excessive weight and dental problems.

Fat

Fat contains more calories per gram (9kcals/g) than carbohydrates (3.75kcals/g). It is therefore not surprising that foods containing a high quantity of fat tend to make one put on weight if eaten in excess. However some amount of fat is essential to a healthy diet as fats provide vitamins A, D, E and K as well as essential fatty acids. It should make up 30 – 35% of the calories we eat.

Eating a moderate, balanced diet is the key to success. Regular exercise is also beneficial. Good Luck.

Weights & Measures

Imperial to Metric

1 ounce (oz) = 28 grams (g)

1 pound (lb) = 454 grams (g)

1 fluid ounce (fl oz) = 30 millilitres (ml)

1 pint = 0.57 litres

Metric to Imperial

100 grams (g) = 3.5 ounces (oz)

1 kilogram (kg) = 2.2 pounds (lb)

100 millilitres (ml) = 3.4 fluid ounces (fl oz)

1 litre = 1.8 pints

Using this book

This book is laid out into sections to make finding foods as easy as possible. Basic, non branded foods are divided into: Breads, Flour, Starches and Grains; Dairy and its products, Fruit, Fish and its products, Fats, Oils and Sauces, Herbs, Meat and Vegetables. There are also lists of common branded foods such as Soups and Tinned Foods. Food is then categorised into common breakfast, lunch and cooked meals. Lunchtime foods display a variety of common salads, sandwiches and snacks. Cooked meals display a wide variety of cuisine from pasta to oriental dishes. We then enter the realm of the 'naughty but nice' sweets and delicacies. There is a section on Drinks and if you like grabbing a quick bite we have counted the calories of five major Fast Food Restaurants. At the end of the book there is an alphabetical listing of the most common foods. This is for easy reference. It will save you having to search through the categories.

The food entries are divided into two categories: per serving and per 100g. The per serving value gives you the values for an individual item such as an apple, or a serving value such as a slice of cake. In this way you can work out the calorie content of each meal. You are also provided with the value for 100g serving. This tool enables you to make comparisons between various foods. All values have been rounded to the nearest gram unless under the value of 5 where the gram has been rounded to the first decimal place.

Please note that the nutritional values are approximations and can be affected by biological and seasonal variations in foods and uncertainty in the dietary database.

This book is intended solely as a guide for following a healthy balanced diet, and is not medical advice. Anyone with specific dietary needs should consult a GP before changing diets.

1
Basic foods

FOOD	SERVING	CARBS (g)	CALS (kcal)	FAT (g)

FLOURS, GRAINS, STARCHES AND BREAD

Flours, Grains

FOOD	SERVING	CARBS (g)	CALS (kcal)	FAT (g)
Arrowroot	1 serving (25g)	23	88	0.0
	Per 100g	90	350	0.1
Barley	1 serving (25g)	18	84	0.4
	Per 100g	72	335	1.4
Bran, wheat	1 serving (25g)	7	52	1.5
	Per 100g	27	206	6
Chapati flour, brown	1 serving (25g)	19	83	0.3
	Per 100g	74	333	1.2
Cornflour	1 serving (25g)	23	89	0.2
	Per 100g	92	354	0.7
Maize	1 serving (25g)	18	88	0.9
	Per 100g	70	352	3.5
Millet	1 serving (25g)	18	90	0.4
	Per 100g	73	358	1.5
Oatmeal, quick cook raw	1 serving (25g)	17	94	2.3
	Per 100g	66	375	9
Rye flour, whole	1 serving (25g)	19	84	0.5
	Per 100g	76	335	2
Semolina	1 serving (25g)	19	84	0.4
	Per 100g	75	335	1.6
Soya flour, full fat	1 serving (25g)	6	112	6
	Per 100g	24	447	24
Soya flour, low fat	1 serving (25g)	7	88	1.8
	Per 100g	28	352	7
Wheat flour white, plain	1 serving (25g)	20	85	0.3
	Per 100g	78	341	1.3
Wheat flour, brown	1 serving (25g)	17	81	0.5
	Per 100g	69	323	1.8
Wheat flour, white, breadmaking	1 serving (25g)	19	85	0.4
	Per 100g	75	341	1.4

FOOD	SERVING	CARBS (g)	CALS (kcal)	FAT (g)
Wheat flour, white, self raising	1 serving (25g)	19	83	0.3
	Per 100g	76	330	1.2
Wheat flour,wholemeal	1 serving (25g)	16	78	0.6
	Per 100g	64	310	2.2

Rice

Basmati, cooked	1 serving (110g)	50	200	0.4
	Per 100g	45	182	0.4
Brown rice, boiled	1 serving (110g)	1	35	2.9
	Per 100g	32	110	1.2
Extra long grain, cooked	1 serving (110g)	64	248	0.6
	Per 100g	58	225	0.5
Savoury rice, cooked	1 serving (110g)	4	29	3.2
	Per 100g	25	135	3.3
Fragrant rice, cooked	1 serving (110g)	42	165	0.3
	Per 100g	38	150	0.3
White rice, easy cook, boiled	1 serving (110g)	1.4	34	2.9
	Per 100g	29	133	1.2
White rice, fried in lard	1 serving (110g)	3.5	28	2.4
	Per 100g	24	130	3

Pasta

Macaroni, raw	1 serving (110g)	79	380	1.7
	Per 100g	72	345	1.5
Macaroni, boiled	1 serving (110g)	18	90	0.6
	Per 100g	16	82	0.5
Noodles, egg, raw	1 serving (110g)	91	425	6.6
	Per 100g	83	386	6
Noodles, egg, boiled	1 serving (110g)	13	77	0.6
	Per 100g	12	70	0.5
Noodles, rice, boiled	1 serving (110g)	28	112	0.6
	Per 100g	25	102	0.5
Noodles, rice, fried	1 serving (150g)	20	240	18.0
	Per 100g	13	160	12

Calorie, Fat & Carbohydrate Counter

FOOD	SERVING	CARBS (g)	CALS (kcal)	FAT (g)
Noodles, buckwheat, boiled	1 serving (110g)	28	112	0.0
	Per 100g	25	102	0
Noodles, quick cook	1 packet (85g)	57	377	14.2
	Per 100g	68	452	17
Noodles, rice, dry	1 portion (110g)	85	391	0.1
	Per 100g	77	355	0.1
Noodles, wheat, fried	1 portion (85g)	53	376	15.0
	Per 100g	63	451	18
Noodles, wheat, steamed	1 portion (85g)	57	271	1.9
	Per 100g	68	325	2.3
Spaghetti, white, raw	1 serving (110g)	78	373	1.8
	Per 100g	71	339	1.6
Spaghetti, white, boiled	1 serving (110g)	70	351	2.6
	Per 100g	64	319	2.4
Spaghetti, wholemeal, raw	1 serving (110g)	31	122	0.9
	Per 100g	28	111	0.8

Pastry

FOOD	SERVING	CARBS (g)	CALS (kcal)	FAT (g)
Pastry, choux	1 serving (30g)	9	105	7
	Per 100g	29	350	24
Pastry, filo	2 sheets (15g)	14	74	0.5
	Per 100g	95	495	3.4
Pastry, flaky	1 serving (50g)	23	290	20
	Per 100g	45	580	40
Pastry, hot water	1 serving (50g)	28	213	10
	Per 100g	55	425	20
Pastry, puff	1 serving (170g)	65	663	43
	Per 100g	38	390	25
Pastry, shortcrust	1 serving (110g)	55	534	32
	Per 100g	50	485	29
Pastry, strudel	1 serving (50g)	23	268	20
	Per 100g	45	535	40
Pastry, suet crust	1 serving (50g)	28	208	11
	Per 100g	55	415	21

FOOD	SERVING	CARBS (g)	CALS (kcal)	FAT (g)
Pastry, wholemeal	1 serving (110g)	50	517	32
	Per 100g	45	470	29

Breads/Rolls/Muffins

FOOD	SERVING	CARBS (g)	CALS (kcal)	FAT (g)
Bagel, egg	1 (about 60g)	33	172	1.5
	Per 100g	55	280	2.4
Bagel, water	1 (about 60g)	33	172	1.5
	Per 100g	55	280	2.5
Biscuit, baking powder, homemade	1 (30g)	14	110	5
	Per 100g	45	365	17
Blueberry, homemade	1 (about 45g)	18	118	4.1
	Per 100g	40	265	9
Bran, homemade	1 (about 45g)	18	110	4.1
	Per 100g	40	240	9
Bread stick, Vienna-type	1 (35g)	21	102	1.1
	Per 100g	60	290	3.2
Brown bread	1 medium slice (about 30g)	13	65	0.6
	Per 100g	45	210	2
Brown bread, toasted	1 medium slice (about 30g)	17	25	0.6
	Per 100g	55	85	1.9
Brown roll, crusty	1 (about 45g)	24	122	1.3
	Per 100g .	55	275	2.9
Brown roll, soft	1 (about 45g)	25	129	1.8
	Per 100g	55	295	4
Chapati, made with fat	1 (about 100g)	45	315	12
	Per 100g	45	315	12
Chapati, made without fat	1 (about 100g)	44	202	1
	Per 100g	44	202	1
Cracked wheat bread	1 slice (about 30g)	14	70	1.8
	Per 100g	45	230	6
Croissant	1 (about 60g)	23	216	12
	Per 100g	38	355	20
Crumpet, toasted	1 (about 45g)	20	90	0.5
	Per 100g	45	195	1

Calorie, Fat & Carbohydrate Counter

FOOD	SERVING	CARBS (g)	CALS (kcal)	FAT (g)
Currant bread	1 slice (about 25g)	13	72	2
	Per 100g	50	290	8
English muffin	1 (about 60g)	32	163	2.5
	Per 100g	55	265	3.9
Focaccia	1 (about 50g)	30	139	1.5
	Per 100g	65	265	3.1
Focaccia, herb & garlic	1 (about 70g)	32	170	1.5
	Per 100g	45	230	2.1
French or Vienna bread	1 slice (35g)	19	96	0.8
	Per 100g	55	275	2.3
Granary bread	1 slice (about 25g)	12	59	0.7
	Per 100g	45	225	2.6
Hamburger roll	1 (about 85g)	42	223	4
	Per 100g	50	275	5
Hot cross buns	1 bun (about 50g)	30	155	3.4
	Per 100g	60	310	7
Italian bread	1 slice (about 30g)	18	88	4
	Per 100g	55	290	14
Malt loaf	1 slice (about 35g)	20	94	0.8
	Per 100g	55	255	2.4
Muffin, 1 medium plain	1 serving (60g)	30	177	8
	Per 100g	50	295	13
Muffin, 1 large	1 serving (100g)	45	270	13
	Per 100g	45	270	13
Muffin, 1 extra large	1 serving (150g)	75	435	20
	Per 100g	50	290	13
Muffin, blueberry	1 serving (150g)	53	338	14
	Per 100g	35	225	9
Muffin, bran	1 serving (190g)	68	513	27
	Per 100g	36	270	14
Muffin, calorie reduced	1 serving (152g)	49	357	18
	Per 100g	32	235	12
Muffin, high fibre	1 serving (63g)	25	154	2
	Per 100g	40	245	3.1

FOOD	SERVING	CARBS (g)	CALS (kcal)	FAT (g)
Muffin, fruit	1 serving (60g)	27	156	1.5
	Per 100g	45	260	2.5
Muffin, spicy fruit topped	1 serving (67g)	30	168	2
	Per 100g	45	250	3
Muffin, white, bread type	1 serving (67g)	30	157	0.9
	Per 100g	45	235	1.4
Muffin, low fat	1 serving (152g)	58	281	2.4
	Per 100g	38	185	1.6
Muffin, mixed berry	1 serving (60g)	39	204	5
	Per 100g	65	340	8
Muffin, apple and sultana	1 serving (60g)	33	195	7
	Per 100g	55	325	12
Muffin, mix, prepared, blueberry and apricot	1 serving (60g)	30	192	7
	Per 100g	50	320	12
Muffin, mix, choc chip	1 serving (60g)	33	219	8
	Per 100g	55	365	13
Naan bread	1 (about 160g)	80	538	20
	Per 100g	50	345	13
Pitta bread (white)	1 pocket (75g)	41	203	0.9
	Per 100g	55	270	1.2
Popover, homemade	1 (about 45g)	11	95	1
	Per 100g	23	220	2.1
Pumpernickel bread	1 slice (about 30g)	18	84	2.7
	Per 100g	60	285	9
Raisin bread	1 slice (about 30g)	14	70	0.4
	Per 100g	45	240	1.4
Roll or bun, homemade	1 (about 35g)	19	118	0.9
	Per 100g	55	350	2.4
Rye bread	1 slice (25g)	11	55	0.5
	Per 100g	45	220	1.8
Sourdough bread	1 slice (30g)	12	74	11
	Per 100g	40	245	38
Wheatgerm loaf	1 slice (25g)	11	59	0.8
	Per 100g	45	235	3.3

Calorie, Fat & Carbohydrate Counter

FOOD	SERVING	CARBS (g)	CALS (kcal)	FAT (g)
White bread, average	1 slice (30g)	15	74	0.6
	Per 100g	50	245	1.9
White bread, french stick	2 stick (40g)	22	110	1.1
	Per 100g	55	275	2.8
White bread, fried in blended oil	1 slice (30g)	14	146	10
	Per 100g	45	485	33
White bread, fried in lard	1 slice (about 30g)	15	151	10
	Per 100g	45	495	33
White bread, Vienna	1slice (25g)	14	65	0.9
	Per 100g	55	260	3.4
White bread, West Indian	1slice (25g)	15	71	0.9
	Per 100g	60	285	3.5
White bread with added fibre	1 slice (40g)	18	82	0.5
	Per 100g	45	205	1.2
White roll, crusty	1 (50g)	30	133	1.1
	Per 100g	60	265	2.2
White roll, soft	1 (50g)	28	135	1.9
	Per 100g	55	270	3.7
Wholemeal bread	1 slice (25g)	10	53	0.6
	Per 100g	40	210	2.4
Wholemeal roll	1 (50g)	23	120	1.6
	Per 100g	45	240	3.1

FOOD	SERVING	CARBS (g)	CALS (kcal)	FAT (g)

DAIRY

Milk

FOOD	SERVING	CARBS	CALS	FAT
Aerosol cream, whipped	1 serving (80ml)	4	236	28
	Per 100g	5	295	35
Buttermilk, dairy	1 glass (200ml)	4	96	4
	Per 100ml	2	48	2
Clotted cream	1 serving (80ml)	2.4	472	46
	Per 100ml	3	590	58
Condensed milk, skimmed, sweetened	1 glass (200ml)	120	530	0.4
	Per 100ml	60	265	0.2
Condensed milk, whole, sweetened	1 glass (200ml)	110	690	20
	Per 100ml	55	345	10
Crème fraiche	1 serving (80ml)	2.8	365	42
	Per 100ml	3.5	456	53
Cultured milk, skimmed	1 glass (200ml)	12	80	0.32
	Per 100ml	6	40	0.2
Dried skimmed milk	1 tsp (15g)	7	52	0.1
	Per 100g	50	345	0.6
Dried skimmed milk, with vegetable fat	1 tsp (15g)	7	75	4
	Per 100g	45	500	27
Evaporated milk, reduced fat	1 glass (200ml)	20	188	4
	Per 100ml	10	94	2
Evaporated milk, whole	1 glass (200ml)	18	300	18
	Per 100ml	9	150	9
Fat-reduced, protein increased	1 glass (200ml)	10.4	96	3.2
	Per 100ml	5.2	48	1.6
Flavoured milk	1 glass (200ml)	22	140	3.2
	Per 100ml	11	70	1.6
Fresh cream, clotted	1 serving (80ml)	1.9	460	52
	Per 100ml	2.4	575	65
Fresh cream, double	1 serving (80ml)	2.2	372	36
	Per 100ml	2.7	465	45

Calorie, Fat & Carbohydrate Counter

FOOD	SERVING	CARBS (g)	CALS (kcal)	FAT (g)
Fresh cream, half, pasteurised	1 serving (80ml)	3.2	120	10
	Per 100ml	4	150	13
Fresh cream, single	1 serving (80ml)	3	156	15
	Per 100ml	3.8	195	19
Fresh cream, soured	1 serving (80ml)	3	156	16
	Per 100ml	3.8	195	20
Fresh cream, whipping	1 serving (80ml)	2.4	296	32
	Per 100ml	3	370	40
Goats milk, pasteurised	1 glass (200ml)	8	120	7
	Per 100ml	4	60	3.6
Imitation cream, Dessert Top	1 serving (80ml)	4.8	224	22
	Per 100ml	6	280	28
Imitation cream, Dream Topping, semi	1 serving (80ml)	9.6	132	10
	Per 100ml	12	165	12
Imitation cream, Dream Topping, whole	1 serving (80ml)	9.6	152	11
	Per 100ml	12	190	14
Imitation cream, Elmlea, double	1 serving (80ml)	2.6	356	40
	Per 100ml	3.3	445	50
Imitation cream, Elmlea, whipping	1 serving (80ml)	2.4	252	26
	Per 100ml	3	315	32
Imitation cream, Emlea, single	1 serving (80ml)	3.2	148	14
	Per 100ml	4	185	18
Imitation cream, Tip Top	1 serving (80ml)	7.2	92	6
	Per 100ml	9	115	7
Low-fat, high calcium	1 glass (200ml)	12.8	104	0.32
	Per 100ml	6.4	52	0.2
Rice milk	1 glass (200ml)	0	132	2.4
	Per 100ml	0	66	1.2
Semi-Skimmed milk, average	1 glass (200ml)	10	90	3
	Per 100ml	5	45	1.5
Semi-Skimmed milk, fortified, plus SMP	1 glass (200ml)	12	100	3.2
	Per 100ml	6	50	1.6
Semi-Skimmed milk, pasteurised	1 glass (200ml)	10	100	3.2
	Per 100ml	5	50	1.6

FOOD	SERVING	CARBS (g)	CALS (kcal)	FAT (g)
Semi-Skimmed milk, UHT, fortified	1 glass (200ml)	10	90	3.4
	Per 100ml	5	45	1.7
Sheep's milk, raw	1 glass (200ml)	10	190	8
	Per 100ml	5	95	4
Skimmed milk, average	1 glass (200ml)	10	64	0.2
	Per 100ml	5	32	0.1
Skimmed milk, fortified, plus SMP	1 glass (200ml)	12	78	0.2
	Per 100ml	6	39	0.1
Skimmed milk, pasteurised	1 glass (200ml)	10	68	0.2
	Per 100ml	5	34	0.1
Skimmed milk, UHT, fortified	1 glass (200ml)	10	70	0.4
	Per 100ml	5	35	0.2
Sour cream, dairy	1 serving (80ml)	3.2	172	15
	Per 100ml	4	215	19
Sour cream, extra light	1 serving (80ml)	4.8	130.	11
	Per 100ml	6	162	14
Sour cream, light	1 serving (80ml)	3.2	158	14
	Per 100ml	4	198	17
Soya milk, flavoured, banana	1 glass (200ml)	20	104	2.4
	Per 100ml	10	52	1.2
Soya milk, flavoured, chocolate hazlenut	1 glass (200ml)	16	128	6.4
	Per 100ml	8	64	3.2
Soya milk, plain	1 glass (200ml)	1.6	64	3.8
	Per 100ml	0.8	32	1.9
Sterilised cream, canned	1 serving (80ml)	3.0	184	19
	Per 100ml	3.7	230	24
UHT cream, canned spray	1 serving (80ml)	2.7	256	26
	Per 100g	3.4	320	33
Whole milk, average	1 glass (200ml)	10	130	8
	Per 100ml	5	65	3.9
Whole milk, sterilised	1 glass (200ml)	10	130	7
	Per 100ml	5	65	3.7
Whole milk, summer	1 glass (200ml)	10	130	8
	Per 100ml	5	65	4

Calorie, Fat & Carbohydrate Counter

FOOD	SERVING	CARBS (g)	CALS (kcal)	FAT (g)
Whole milk, winter	1 glass (200ml)	10	130	8
	Per 100ml	5	65	3.9

Cheese

FOOD	SERVING	CARBS (g)	CALS (kcal)	FAT (g)
American	1 portion (85g)	1.4	293	26
	Per 100g	1.7	345	31
Blue	1 portion (85g)	2	268	23
	Per 100g	2.3	315	27
Blue brie	1 portion (85g)	0	357	38
	Per 100g	0	420	45
Blue castello	1 portion (85g)	0	302	27
	Per 100g	0	355	32
Blue vein	1 portion (85g)	0	306	27
	Per 100g	0	360	32
Brick	1 portion (85g)	2.3	298	22
	Per 100g	2.7	350	26
Brie	1 portion (85g)	0.3	259	21
	Per 100g	0.3	305	25
Bocconcini	1 portion (85g)	0	221	20
	Per 100g	0	260	24
Camembert	1 portion (85g)	0.3	230	20
	Per 100g	0.3	270	24
Canola, mild	1 portion (85g)	0	259	19
	Per 100g	0	305	22
Caraway	1 portion (85g)	2.6	285	22
	Per 100g	3	335	26
Cheddar	1 portion (85g)	1.1	327	26
	Per 100g	1.3	385	30
Cheddar, low fat	1 portion (85g)	0	264	20
	Per 100g	0	310	24
Cheshire	1 portion (85g)	0	315	27
	Per 100g	0	370	32
Colby	1 portion (85g)	2	319	26
	Per 100g	2.3	375	31

FOOD	SERVING	CARBS (g)	CALS (kcal)	FAT (g)
Cottage with pineapple, low fat	1 portion (85g)	9	77	0
	Per 100g	10	90	0
Cream cheese	1 portion (85g)	2	268	27
	Per 100g	2.3	315	32
Cream, fruit	1 portion (85g)	0	225	21
	Per 100g	0	265	25
Cream, light	1 portion (85g)	2.8	132	14
	Per 100g	3.3	155	16
Creamed cottage	1 portion (85g)	1.4	68	2.9
	Per 100g	1.6	80	3.4
Creamed cottage, low fat	1 portion (85g)	2.8	55	1.4
	Per 100g	3.3	65	1.7
Double Gloucester	1 portion (85g)	0	353	29
	Per 100g	0	415	34
Emmental	1 portion (85g)	0	306	26
	Per 100g	0	360	30
Edam	1 portion (85g)	1.1	268	23
	Per 100g	1.3	315	27
Feta	1 portion (85g)	3.4	208	16
	Per 100g	4	245	19
Fontina	1 portion (85g)	1	293	26
	Per 100g	1.2	345	31
Gouda	1 portion (85g)	1.7	293	22
	Per 100g	2	345	26
Gruyere	1 portion (85g)	0.3	336	25
	Per 100g	0.3	395	29
Goat's	1 portion (85g)	1.4	162	14
	Per 100g	1.6	190	17
Halloumi	1 portion (85g)	0	200	14
	Per 100g	0	235	17
Havarti	1 portion (85g)	0	353	30
	Per 100g	0	415	35
Jarlsberg	1 portion (85g)	0	332	25
	Per 100g	0	390	29

Calorie, Fat & Carbohydrate Counter

FOOD	SERVING	CARBS (g)	CALS (kcal)	FAT (g)
Jarlsberg lite	1 portion (85g)	0	225	14
	Per 100g	0	265	17
Lancashire	1 portion (85g)	0	310	28
	Per 100g	0	365	33
Leicester	1 portion (85g)	0	344	27
	Per 100g	0	405	32
Monterey Jack	1 portion (85g)	0.6	298	26
	Per 100g	0.7	350	31
Mozzarella, part-skim	1 portion (85g)	2.3	191	14
	Per 100g	2.7	225	17
Mozzarella, whole-milk	1 portion (85g)	1.7	213	17
	Per 100g	2	250	20
Muenster	1 portion (85g)	0.9	281	22
	Per 100g	1	330	26
Neufchatel	1 portion (85g)	2.1	213	19
	Per 100g	2.5	250	22
Parmesan, grated	1 portion (85g)	0.6	349	25
	Per 100g	0.7	410	29
Provolone	1 portion (85g)	1.7	281	21
	Per 100g	2	330	25
Romano, grated	1 portion (85g)	0.6	55	4.3
	Per 100g	0.7	65	5
Roquefort	1 portion (85g)	1.7	281	25
	Per 100g	2	330	29
Swiss	1 portion (85g)	2.8	306	22
	Per 100g	3.3	360	26
Sheep's milk, fresh	1 portion (85g)	0	255	20
	Per 100g	0	300	24
Soya	1 portion (85g)	0	255	22
	Per 100g	0	300	26
Stilton	1 portion (85g)	0	323	29
	Per 100g	0	380	34
Wensleydale	1 portion (85g)	0	310	26
	Per 100g	0	365	31

FOOD	SERVING	CARBS (g)	CALS (kcal)	FAT (g)
Yogurt cheese, low-fat	1 portion (85g)	7	81	1.6
	Per 100g	8	95	1.9

Eggs

FOOD	SERVING	CARBS (g)	CALS (kcal)	FAT (g)
Chicken poached	1 serving (55g)	0	83	6
	Per 100g	0	150	11
Chicken scrambled with milk	1 serving (55g)	0.3	135	13
	Per 100g	0.6	245	23
Chicken, boiled	1 serving (25g)	0	36	2.8
	Per 100g	0	145	11
Chicken, fried in vegetable oil	1 serving (55g)	0	96	7
	Per 100g	0	175	13
Chicken, white, raw	1 serving (25g)	0	9	0
	Per 100g	0	37	0
Chicken, whole, raw	1 medium (55g)	0	74	6
	Per 100g	0	135	10
Chicken, yolk, raw	1 serving (25g)	0	84	8
	Per 100g	0	335	30
Duck, boiled	1 large (65g)	tr	111	8
	Per 100g	tr	170	13
Duck, whole raw	1 medium (55g)	0	85	7
	Per 100g	0	155	12
Egg fried rice	1 serving (100g)	25	210	11
	Per 100g	25	210	11
Meringue	1 serving (25g)	25	93	0
	Per 100g	100	370	0
Meringue with cream	1 serving (25g)	10	91	6
	Per 100g	40	365	23
Omelette, cheese	1 serving (100g)	0	255	23
	Per 100g	0	255	23
Omelette, plain	1 serving (100g)	0	185	16
	Per 100g	0	185	16
Quail, raw	1 (10g)	0	17	1
	Per 100g	0	165	10

Calorie, Fat & Carbohydrate Counter

FOOD	SERVING	CARBS (g)	CALS (kcal)	FAT (g)
Quiche, cheese and egg	1 serving (100g)	17	305	23
	Per 100g	17	305	23
Quiche, cheese, egg, wholemeal	1 serving (100g)	16	315	21
	Per 100g	16	315	21
Scotch eggs, retail	1 serving (100g)	13	255	16
	Per 100g	13	255	16
Turkey, raw	1 (80g)	tr	124	10
	Per 100g	tr	155	13

Ice cream

FOOD	SERVING	CARBS (g)	CALS (kcal)	FAT (g)
Arctic roll	1 serving (120g)	41	246	8
	Per 100g	34	205	7
Choc ice	1 serving (120g)	32	330	22
	Per 100g	27	275	18
Chocolate sundae	1 serving (120g)	40	348	18
	Per 100g	33	290	15
Cornetto	1 serving (120g)	43	306	16
	Per 100g	36	255	13
Frozen ice cream desserts	1 serving (120g)	26	264	16
	Per 100g	22	220	13
Ice cream, flavoured	1 serving (120g)	31	222	10
	Per 100g	26	185	8
Ice cream wafers	1 wafer (15g)	11	53	0.1
	Per 100g	75	355	0.7
Ice cream, cone, chocolate	1 serving (70g)	23	228	13
	Per 100g	33	325	18
Ice cream, cone, vanilla	1 serving (70g)	32	289	16
	Per 100g	45	405	23
Ice cream, cone, single plain wafer type	1 serving (70g)	4	18	0
	Per 100g	6	26	0
Ice cream, cone, sugar	1 serving (15g)	8	41	0.5
	Per 100g	55	275	3.3
Ice cream, cone, waffle	1 serving (10g)	3.4	15	0
	Per 100g	34	150	0

FOOD	SERVING	CARBS (g)	CALS (kcal)	FAT (g)
Ice cream, dairy, vanilla	1 serving (120g)	29	240	12
	Per 100g	24	200	10
Ice cream, double chocolate	1 serving (120g)	48	492	29
	Per 100g	40	410	24
Ice cream, lemon	1 serving (120g)	47	330	16
	Per 100g	39	275	13
Ice cream, light and creamy vanilla	1 serving (120g)	32	168	3
	Per 100g	27	140	2.8
Ice cream, mango	1 serving (120g)	44	36	17
	Per 100g	37	305	14
Ice cream, natural vanilla	1 serving (120g)	20	210	13
	Per 100g	17	175	11
Ice cream, original vanilla	1 serving (120g)	20	192	11
	Per 100g	17	160	9
Ice cream, raspberry	1 serving (120g)	40	252	8
	Per 100g	33	210	7
Ice cream, soft serve	1 serving (120g)	48	300	10
	Per 100g	40	250	8
Ice cream, stick, belgian, chocolate coated	1 serving (65g)	42	429	26
	Per 100g	65	660	40
Ice cream, stick, chocolate flavoured	1 serving (50g)	20	120	3.5
	Per 100g	40	240	7
Ice cream, stick, vanilla, chocolate covered	1 serving (52g)	20	239	17
	Per 100g	39	460	33
Ice cream, tub, strawberries and cream	1 tub (55g)	25	198	11
	Per 100g	45	360	20
Ice cream, tub, chocolate	1 tub (55g)	9	91	6
	Per 100g	17	165	10
Ice cream, tub, cookies and fudge	1 tub (55g)	15	204	17
	Per 100g	27	370	30
Ice cream, tub, fruit cream	1 tub (55g)	10	96	5
	Per 100g	18	175	9
Ice cream, tub, original extra creamy vanilla	1 tub (55g)	10	99	6
	Per 100g	19	180	10

Calorie, Fat & Carbohydrate Counter

FOOD	SERVING	CARBS (g)	CALS (kcal)	FAT (g)
Ice cream, tub, vanilla	1 tub (55g)	21	182	9
	Per 100g	38	330	17
Ice cream, tub, vanilla light	1 tub (55g)	12	85	2.8
	Per 100g	21	155	5
Ice cream, vienetta style, vanilla	1 serving (55g)	13	124	10
	Per 100g	24	225	18
Ice cream, vienetta style, chocolate	1 serving (55g)	13	132	9
	Per 100g	24	240	16
Ice cream,vienetta style, toffee	1 serving (55g)	13	129	10
	Per 100g	23	235	18
Ice-cream, non-dairy, flavoured	1 serving (120g)	28	198	8
	Per 100g	23	165	7
Ice-cream, non-dairy, mixed	1 serving (120g)	30	222	10
	Per 100g	25	185	8
Ice-ream, non-dairy, vanilla	1 serving (120g)	28	216	11
	Per 100g	23	180	9
Sorbet, lemon	1 serving (120g)	40	162	0
	Per 100g	33	135	0

Ice cream – brands

FOOD	SERVING	CARBS (g)	CALS (kcal)	FAT (g)
Banoffee Fudge Ice Cream (Sainsbury's)	1/8 tub (67g)	19	119	4
	Per 100g	29	178	6
Caramel Cone Ice Cream (Haagen-Dazs)	1 scoop (85g)	22	258	17
	Per 100g	26	303	20
Caramel Ice Cream Bar (Cadbury's)	1 bar (64g)	20	188	11
	Per 100g	32	294	17
Chocolate Fudge Swirl Ice Cream (Haagen-Dazs)	1 scoop (85g)	22	235	14
	Per 100g	26	276	17
Chocolate Ice Cream Organic (Iceland)	1 scoop (85g)	25	177	7
	Per 100g	29	208	8
Chocolate Ice Cream Organic (M&S)	1 scoop (85g)	20	217	14
	Per 100g	24	255	16
Chocolate Ice Cream (Thorntons)	1 scoop (85g)	21	202	11
	Per 100g	25	238	13

FOOD	SERVING	CARBS (g)	CALS (kcal)	FAT (g)
Ice Cream Gateau Cassatta Siciliana (M&S)	1 serving (93g)	30	263	15
	Per 100g	32	283	16
Magic Maple Ice Cream (M&S)	1 ice cream (93g)	36	259	11
	Per 100g	39	278	12
Strawberry & Cream Organic (Sainsbury's)	1 serving (100g)	23	193	10
	Per 100g	23	193	10
Strawberry & Vanilla Cones (Sainsbury's)	1 cone (62g)	23	153	6
	Per 100g	37	247	10
Strawberry & Vanilla Ice Lolly Fat Free (Iceland)	1 lolly (92g)	22	98	0.4
	Per 100g	24	107	0.4
Strawberry Cheesecake Ice Cream (Haagen-Dazs)	1 scoop (85g)	23	226	14
	Per 100g	27	266	16
Strawberry Sorbet (M&S)	1 scoop (85g)	20	81	0.1
	Per 100g	23	95	0.1
Strawberry Split (Co-Op)	1 lolly (55g)	10	62	2
	Per 100g	19	112	3.7
Toffee Crème Ice Cream (Haagen-Dazs)	1 scoop (85g)	23	225	14
	Per 100g	27	265	16
Toffee Ice Cream Deliciously Dairy (Co-Op)	1 scoop (85g)	18	136	6
	Per 100g	21	160	7
Toffee Ice Cream (Thorntons)	1 scoop (85g)	21	185	10
	Per 100g	25	218	12
Viennetta Chocolate (Wall's)	1 serving (55g)	13	138	8
	Per 100g	24	250	15

Yogurts

FOOD	SERVING	CARBS (g)	CALS (kcal)	FAT (g)
Yogurt, bio type, low fat, honey	1 serving (100g)	13	100	3
	Per 100g	13	100	3
Yogurt, black cherry, with live cultures	1 serving (100g)	17	104	4
	Per 100g	17	104	4
Yogurt, drinking, apricot	1 serving (250g)	31	190	5
	Per 100g	12	76	2
Yogurt, drinking	1 serving (100g)	13	81	1
	Per 100g	13	81	1

Calorie, Fat & Carbohydrate Counter

FOOD	SERVING	CARBS (g)	CALS (kcal)	FAT (g)
Yogurt, drinking, swiss type, vanilla	1 serving (250g)	32	184	5
	Per 100g	13	74	2
Yogurt, drinking, vitamin enriched	1 serving (100g)	24	139	5
	Per 100g	24	139	5
Yogurt, drinking, fruit	1 serving (250g)	32	190	5
	Per 100g	13	76	2
Yogurt, frozen, fruit	1 serving (250g)	20	132	5
	Per 100g	8	53	2
Yogurt, frozen, fruit, yogurt stick, raspberry	1 serving (250g)	20	132	5
	Per 100g	8	53	2
Yogurt, low fat, flavoured	1 serving (100g)	22	83	0
	Per 100g	22	83	0
Yoplait, Wildlife choobs	1 carton (113g)	16	124	8.9
	Per 100g	14	110	8
Yoplait, Frubes	1 carton (100g)	24	192	8
	Per 100g	24	192	8
Yoplait, Petit filous	1 carton (100g)	15	114	2.9
	Per 100g	15	114	2.9
Yoplait, Yo-to-go	1 carton (100g)	15	95	2.4
	Per 100g	15	95	2.4
Banana choco flakes	1 carton (150g)	34	218	6
	Per 100g	23	145	4
Coco pops	1 carton (150g)	29	180	5
	Per 100g	19	120	3.1
Frosties	1 carton (150g)	30	185	4
	Per 100g	20	123	2.9
Toffee hoops	1 carton (150g)	33	242	9
	Per 100g	22	161	6

Fromage frais

FOOD	SERVING	CARBS (g)	CALS (kcal)	FAT (g)
Yoplait, apricot, mango and vanilla	1 carton (124g)	20	122	2
	Per 100g	16	98	1.6
Yoplait, black cherry	1 carton (125g)	20	134	2
	Per 100g	16	107	1.6

FOOD	SERVING	CARBS (g)	CALS (kcal)	FAT (g)
Yoplait, blackberry, apple and vanilla	1 carton (125g)	22	126	2
	Per 100g	17	101	1.6
Yoplait, nectarine, orange and vanilla	1 carton (124g)	21	123	2
	Per 100g	17	99	1.6
Yoplait, peach and apricot	1 carton (125g)	18	128	2
	Per 100g	14	102	1.6
Yoplait, strawberry	1 carton (100g)	6	48	0.1
	Per 100g	6	48	0.1
Yoplait, strawberry and vanilla	1 carton (124g)	21	123	2
	Per 100g	17	99	1.6
Yoplait, summer fruits	1 carton (125g)	18	128	2
	Per 100g	14	102	1.6

Ski low fat yogurts

FOOD	SERVING	CARBS (g)	CALS (kcal)	FAT (g)
Ski light, blackberry and raspberry	1 carton (126g)	9	67	0.3
	Per 100g	7	53	0.2
Ski light, peach and pineapple	1 carton (130g)	10	70	0.1
	Per 100g	8	54	0.1
Ski light, red cherry	1 carton (127g)	9	61	0.3
	Per 100g	7	48	0.2
Ski light, strawberry	1 carton (127g)	9	61	0.3
	Per 100g	7	48	0.2
Ski low fat yogurts, apricot and mango	1 carton (126g)	21	127	2.3
	Per 100g	16	101	1.8
Ski low fat yogurts, black cherry	1 carton (126g)	21	130	2.3
	Per 100g	17	103	1.8
Ski low fat yogurts, lemon	1 carton (125g)	20	130	2.5
	Per 100g	16	104	2
Ski low fat yogurts, orange and guava	1 carton (125g)	20	128	2.4
	Per 100g	16	102	1.9
Ski low fat yogurts, orange and lemon	1 carton (125g)	20	128	2.4
	Per 100g	16	102	1.9
Ski low fat yogurts, passionfruit and peach	1 carton (125g)	21	129	2.4
	Per 100g	16	103	1.9

Calorie, Fat & Carbohydrate Counter

FOOD	SERVING	CARBS (g)	CALS (kcal)	FAT (g)
Ski low fat yogurts, peach	1 carton (126g)	21	127	2.3
	Per 100g	16	101	1.8
Ski low fat yogurts, pineapple and grapefruit	1 carton (126g)	21	127	2.3
	Per 100g	16	101	1.8
Ski low fat yogurts, pineapple and papaya	1 carton (126g)	21	127	2.3
	Per 100g	16	101	1.8
Ski low fat yogurts, pink grapefruit	1 carton (126g)	21	127	2.3
	Per 100g	16	101	1.8
Ski low fat yogurts, raspberry	1 carton (125g)	20	125	2.4
	Per 100g	16	100	1.9
Ski low fat yogurts, strawberry	1 carton (125g)	20	124	2.3
	Per 100g	16	99	1.8

Benecol Yogurt (low fat yogurt)

Benecol low fat bio yogurt, apricot	1 carton (126g)	18	98	0.8
	Per 100g	14	78	0.6
Benecol low fat bio yogurt, cherry	1 carton (126g)	19	101	0.8
	Per 100g	15	80	0.6
Benecol low fat bio yogurt, raspberry	1 carton (125g)	18	99	0.8
	Per 100g	15	79	0.6
Benecol low fat bio yogurt, strawberry	1 carton (126g)	18	98	0.8
	Per 100g	15	78	0.6

St. Ivel Shape – simply berries (fat free)

Blackberry and raspberry	1 carton (118g)	7	53	0.1
	Per 100g	6	45	0.1
Cranberry and blackcurrant	1 carton (120g)	7	54	0.1
	Per 100g	6	45	0.1
Red cherries	1 carton (119g)	8	57	0.1
	Per 100g	6	48	0.1
Strawberry	1 carton (119g)	7	56	0.1
	Per 100g	6	47	0.1

FOOD	SERVING	CARBS (g)	CALS (kcal)	FAT (g)
Tesco range				
Bio yogurt	1 carton (450g)	261	212	0.9
	Per 100g	58	47	0.2
Bio yogurt – apricot	1 carton (124g)	7	51	0.2
	Per 100g	5	41	0.2
Bio yogurt – mango	1 carton (124g)	7	51	0.2
	Per 100g	5	41	0.2
Bio yogurt – morello cherry	1 carton (124g)	7	51	0.2
	Per 100g	5	41	0.2
Bio yogurt – nectarine and orange	1 carton (131g)	7	51	0.3
	Per 100g	6	39	0.2
Bio yogurt – peach and vanilla	1 carton (124g)	7	51	0.2
	Per 100g	5	41	0.2
Bio yogurt – raspberry	1 carton (120g)	6	49	0.2
	Per 100g	5	41	0.2
Bio yogurt – strawberry	1 carton (125g)	7	50	0.3
	Per 100g	5	40	0.2
Bio yogurt – strawberry and raspberry	1 carton (125g)	7	50	0.3
	Per 100g	5	40	0.2
Fig banana and muesli	1 carton (170g)	34	207	5
	Per 100g	20	122	2.9
Finest – Bourbon vanilla	1 carton (150g)	29	227	10
	Per 100g	19	151	7
Finest – champagne and rhubarb	1 carton (152g)	26	213	10
	Per 100g	17	140	7
Finest – Devonshire style fudge	1 carton (150g)	34	281	14
	Per 100g	22	187	9
Finest – lemon curd	1 carton (150g)	30	272	14
	Per 100g	20	181	9
Finest – natural	1 carton (150g)	10	120	6
	Per 100g	7	80	3.7
Finest – Scottish raspberry	1 carton (150g)	28	227	10
	Per 100g	19	151	7

Calorie, Fat & Carbohydrate Counter

FOOD	SERVING	CARBS (g)	CALS (kcal)	FAT (g)
Finest – strawberries and cream	1 carton (150g)	28	227	10
	Per 100g	19	151	7
Finest – Swiss black cherry	1 carton (150g)	24	210	10
	Per 100g	16	140	7
Honey and muesli breakfast break	1 carton (170g)	34	207	5
	Per 100g	20	122	2.7
Italian style – crème caramel	1 carton (100g)	22	114	1.6
	Per 100g	22	114	1.6
Italian style – tiramisu	1 carton (100g)	33	266	12
	Per 100g	33	266	12
Low fat yogurt – apricot	1 carton (125g)	17	111	2.1
	Per 100g	13	89	1.7
Low fat yogurt – banana	1 carton (125g)	18	114	2.1
	Per 100g	14	91	1.7
Low fat yogurt – blackcurrant	1 carton (125g)	17	110	2.1
	Per 100g	13	88	1.7
Low fat yogurt – cherry	1 carton (125g)	17	110	2.1
	Per 100g	13	88	1.7
Low fat yogurt – gooseberry	1 carton (125g)	16	106	2.1
	Per 100g	13	85	1.7
Low fat yogurt – hazelnut	1 carton (125g)	20	133	3.4
	Per 100g	16	106	2.7
Low fat yogurt – mango	1 carton (125g)	17	111	2.1
	Per 100g	14	89	1.7
Low fat yogurt – orange	1 carton (125g)	17	111	2.1
	Per 100g	14	89	1.7
Low fat yogurt – pineapple	1 carton (125g)	17	111	2.1
	Per 100g	13	89	1.7
Low fat yogurt – raspberry	1 carton (125g)	16	109	2.1
	Per 100g	13	87	1.7
Low fat yogurt – rhubarb	1 carton (125g)	16	106	2.1
	Per 100g	12	85	1.7
Low fat yogurt – strawberry	1 carton (125g)	17	110	2
	Per 100g	14	88	1.6

FOOD	SERVING	CARBS (g)	CALS (kcal)	FAT (g)
Low fat yogurt – toffee	1 carton (125g)	24	143	2.3
	Per 100g	20	114	1.8
Melon breakfast	1 carton (450g)	63	365	5
	Per 100g	14	81	1.2
Natural fromage frais	1 carton (450g)	15	207	0.9
	Per 100g	3.3	46	0.2
Natural – greek style	1 carton (500g)	33	715	55
	Per 100g	7	143	11
Natural – greek style – low fat	1 carton (450g)	36	455	23
	Per 100g	8	101	5
Natural – low fat	1 carton (450g)	63	365	5
	Per 100g	14	81	1.1
Pink grapefruit and muesli	1 carton (170g)	34	204	4
	Per 100g	20	120	2.6
Vanilla yogurt light	1 carton (200g)	17	106	0.2
	Per 100g	8	53	0.1
West country – banana	1 carton (125g)	25	161	5
	Per 100g	20	129	3.7
West country – campina delice	1 carton (100g)	19	136	5
	Per 100g	19	136	5
West country – cappuccino	1 carton (125g)	29	184	5
	Per 100g	24	147	4
West country – toffee and fudge	1 carton (125g)	28	190	6
	Per 100g	22	152	5
West country – vanilla	1 carton (12g)	3	19	1
	Per 100g	24	157	5

Heinz Weight Watchers' yogurts

FOOD	SERVING	CARBS (g)	CALS (kcal)	FAT (g)
Low fat yoplait black cherry	1 carton (120g)	8	55	0.1
	Per 100g	7	46	0.1
Low fat yoplait peach	1 carton (116g)	8	52	0.1
	Per 100g	7	45	0.1
Low fat yoplait raspberry	1 carton (120g)	7	49	0.1
	Per 100g	6	41	0.1

Calorie, Fat & Carbohydrate Counter

FOOD	SERVING	CARBS (g)	CALS (kcal)	FAT (g)
Low fat yoplait strawberry	1 carton (121g)	8	52	0.1
	Per 100g	6	43	0.1
Low fat yoplait toffee	1 carton (121g)	8	52	0.1
	Per 100g	6	43	0.1
Low fat yoplait vanilla	1 carton (122g)	7	50	0.1
	Per 100g	6	41	0.1

Other

Bio activa low fat natural	1 carton (540g)	33	324	10
	Per 100g	6	60	1.9
Munch bunch fromage pot shots	1 carton (40g)	6	50	1.6
	Per 100g	15	124	4
Onken natural bio pot	1 carton (500g)	27	350	19
	Per 100g	5	70	3.7

Tesco dessert range

Belgian chocolate and orange mousse	1 carton (300g)	84	771	42
	Per 100g	28	257	14
Cherries and chocolate fromage frais	1 carton (165g)	33	299	15
	Per 100g	20	181	9
Chocolate brownie sundae	1 carton (150g)	45	564	41
	Per 100g	30	376	27
Chocolate heaven fromage frais	1 carton (176g)	39	396	23
	Per 100g	22	225	13
Chocolate supreme	1 carton (150g)	27	251	14
	Per 100g	18	167	9
Fruit cocktail trifle	1 carton (113g)	22	175	9
	Per 100g	20	155	8
Peach melba sundae	1 carton (150g)	33	261	13
	Per 100g	22	174	9
Rainforest bliss fromage frais	1 carton (167g)	33	279	13
	Per 100g	20	167	8
Raspberry trifle	1 carton (113g)	21	172	9
	Per 100g	19	152	8

Dairy

FOOD	SERVING	CARBS (g)	CALS (kcal)	FAT (g)
Strawberry cheesecake	1 carton (100g)	325	254	12
	Per 100g	33	254	12
Strawberry trifle	1 carton (94g)	17	141	7
	Per 100g	18	150	8
Summer fruit pavlova fromage frais	1 carton (167g)	37	245	7
	Per 100g	22	147	4
Summer fruit pavlova mousse	1 carton (300g)	69	525	25
	Per 100g	23	175	8
Toffee sundae	1 carton (150g)	43	533	39
	Per 100g	29	355	26
Tropical sundae	1 carton (150g)	34	473	36
	Per 100g	23	315	24

Onken mousse

FOOD	SERVING	CARBS (g)	CALS (kcal)	FAT (g)
Onken mousse, peaches	1 carton (150g)	23	215	10
	Per 100g	15	143	7
Onken mousse, strawberry	1 carton (150g)	22	212	10
	Per 100g	15	141	7
Onken mousse, lite lemon	1 carton (150g)	27	156	2.3
	Per 100g	18	104	1.5

Cadbury's

FOOD	SERVING	CARBS (g)	CALS (kcal)	FAT (g)
Cadbury's Flake mousse	1 carton (100g)	29	266	14
	Per 100g	29	266	14
Cadbury's Mousse original	1 carton (100g)	26	192	7
	Per 100g	26	192	7
Cadbury's Trifle	1 carton (100g)	24	276	18
	Per 100g	24	276	18

Muller

FOOD	SERVING	CARBS (g)	CALS (kcal)	FAT (g)
Muller – desserts, Mississippi mud pie	1 carton (150g)	39	254	8
	Per 100g	26	169	5
Muller – desserts, rhubarb crumble	1 carton (150g)	33	222	8
	Per 100g	22	148	5

Calorie, Fat & Carbohydrate Counter

FOOD	SERVING	CARBS (g)	CALS (kcal)	FAT (g)
Muller – desserts, strawberry crumble	1 carton (150g)	33	222	8
	Per 100g	22	148	5
Muller – fruit crunch, rum and raisin	1 carton (150g)	33	219	7
	Per 100g	22	146	5
Muller – fruit crunch, strawberry and orange	1 carton (150g)	34	218	6
	Per 100g	23	145	4
Muller fruit corners, blackberry and raspberry	1 carton (175g)	26	193	7
	Per 100g	15	110	3.9
Muller fruit corners, blueberry	1 carton (175g)	27	196	7
	Per 100g	16	112	3.9
Muller fruit corners, peach and apricot	1 carton (175g)	26	193	7
	Per 100g	15	110	3.9
Muller fruit corners, red cherries	1 carton (175g)	26	193	7
	Per 100g	15	110	3.9
Muller fruit corners, strawberry	1 carton (175g)	30	207	7
	Per 100g	17	118	3.9
Muller light peach and maracuya	1 carton (200g)	16	100	0.2
	Per 100g	8	50	0.1
Muller light summer fruit mousse	1 carton (149g)	28	143	10
	Per 100g	19	96	6
Muller light yogurt banana	1 carton (200g)	17	106	0.2
	Per 100g	9	53	0.1
Muller light yogurt cherry	1 carton (200g)	16	100	0.2
	Per 100g	8	50	0.1
Muller light yogurt chocolate	1 carton (200g)	16	108	0.6
	Per 100g	8	54	0.3
Muller light yogurt country berries	1 carton (200g)	17	104	0.2
	Per 100g	8	52	0.1
Muller light yogurt lemon and lime	1 carton (200g)	16	106	0.2
	Per 100g	8	53	0.1
Muller light yogurt pineapple peach	1 carton (200g)	17	106	0.2
	Per 100g	9	53	0.1
Muller light yogurt strawberry	1 carton (200g)	17	106	0.2
	Per 100g	9	53	0.1

FOOD	SERVING	CARBS (g)	CALS (kcal)	FAT (g)
Muller light yogurt toffee	1 carton (200g)	17	106	0.2
	Per 100g	9	53	0.1
Muller rice raspberry	1 carton (200g)	40	228	5
	Per 100g	20	114	2.3
Muller rice strawberry	1 carton (200g)	40	230	5
	Per 100g	20	115	2.4
Muller rice vanilla custard	1 carton (200g)	44	250	5
	Per 100g	22	125	2.6
Muller thick and cream smooth original	1 carton (500g)	57	545	25
	Per 100g	11	109	5
Muller thick and cream smooth strawberry	1 carton (500g)	84	560	16
	Per 100g	17	112	3.2
Muller vitality probiotic raspberry	1 carton (200g)	31	194	3.6
	Per 100g	15	97	1.8

Calorie, Fat & Carbohydrate Counter

FOOD	SERVING	CARBS (g)	CALS (kcal)	FAT (g)
FRUIT				
Apples, cooking stewed with sugar	1 serving (120g)	23	90	0.1
	Per 100g	19	75	0.1
Apples, cooking stewed without sugar	1 serving (120g)	10	38	0.1
	Per 100g	8	32	0.1
Apples, eating, raw, peeled	1 average (120g)	11	44	0.1
	Per 100g	9	37	0.1
Apples, eating, raw, unpeeled	1 average (120g)	7	31	0.1
	Per 100g	6	26	0.1
Apricot, canned in juice	1 average (120g)	10	42	0.1
	Per 100g	8	35	0.1
Apricot, canned in syrup	1 average (120g)	18	78	0.1
	Per 100g	15	65	0.1
Apricots	3 raw average (110g)	8	35	0.1
	Per 100g	7	32	0.1
Apricots, Dried	3 whole average (50g)	19	80	0.3
	Per 100g	37	160	0.6
Avocado, average	1 average medium (120g)	1.6	162	17
	Per 100g	1.3	135	14
Bananas	1 average, peeled (140g)	32	133	0.4
	Per 100g	23	95	0.3
Blackberries, raw	1 serving (60g)	3	16	0.1
	Per 100g	5	26	0.2
Blackcurrants, raw	1 serving (60g)	4	16	tr
	Per 100g	7	27	tr
Cherries, canned in syrup	1 serving (120g)	22	84	tr
	Per 100g	18	70	tr
Cherries, glace	6 (30g)	20	77	tr
	Per 100g	65	255	tr
Cherries, raw	1 serving (120g)	13	60	0.1
	Per 100g	11	50	0.1
Cherries, raw, weighed with stones	1 serving (160g)	16	62	0.2
	Per 100g	10	39	0.1

FOOD	SERVING	CARBS (g)	CALS (kcal)	FAT (g)
Cherry pie filling	1 serving (160g)	35	136	tr
	Per 100g	22	85	tr
Clementines, raw	1 average (120g)	11	43	0.1
	Per 100g	9	36	0.1
Currants	1 serving (70g)	49	193	0.3
	Per 100g	70	275	0.4
Damsons, raw with stones	1 serving (60g)	5	20	tr
	Per 100g	9	34	tr
Dates, dried with stones	6 average (60g)	33	132	0.1
	Per 100g	55	220	0.2
Dates, raw with stones	1 serving (60g)	16	63	0.1
	Per 100g	27	105	0.1
Figs, dried	5 average (80g)	44	180	1.3
	Per 100g	55	225	1.6
Figs, ready to eat	1 average medium (90g)	45	194	1.3
	Per 100g	50	215	1.4
Fruit cocktail, canned in juice	1 serving (120g)	8	35	tr
	Per 100g	7	29	tr
Fruit cocktail, canned in syrup	1 serving (120g)	18	72	tr
	Per 100g	15	60	tr
Fruit pie filling	1 serving (160g)	30	120	tr
	Per 100g	19	75	tr
Fruit salad, homemade	1 serving (160g)	22	88	0.2
	Per 100g	14	55	0.1
Gooseberries, stewed without sugar	1 serving (120g)	3	19	0.4
	Per 100g	2.5	16	0.3
Gooseberries, canned in syrup	1 serving (120g)	23	90	0.2
	Per 100g	19	75	0.2
Gooseberries, raw	1 serving (120g)	3.7	22	0.5
	Per 100g	3.1	18	0.4
Gooseberries, stewed with sugar	1 serving (120g)	16	60	0.4
	Per 100g	13	50	0.3
Grapefruit canned in juice	1 serving (120g)	8	35	tr
	Per 100g	7	29	tr

Calorie, Fat & Carbohydrate Counter

FOOD	SERVING	CARBS (g)	CALS (kcal)	FAT (g)
Grapefruit canned in syrup	1 serving (120g)	19	72	tr
	Per 100g	16	60	tr
Grapefruit, raw weighed with pips and peel	1/2 grapefruit (250g)	13	48	0.3
	Per 100g	5	19	0.1
Grapefruit, raw, peeled	1/2 grapefruit (130g)	9	38	0.1
	Per 100g	7	29	0.1
Grapes	1 serving (120g)	18	72	0.1
	Per 100g	15	60	0.1
Grapes, with pips	1 serving (120g)	18	72	0.1
	Per 100g	15	60	0.1
Guava weighed with skin and pips	1medium (110g)	6	28	0.6
	Per 100g	5	25	0.5
Guava, canned in syrup	1 serving (120g)	18	72	tr
	Per 100g	15	60	tr
Guava, raw	1 serving (120g)	6	32	0.6
	Per 100g	5	27	0.5
Kiwi fruit, peeled	1 small (80g)	9	40	0.4
	Per 100g	11	50	0.5
Kiwi fruit, weighed with skin	1 medium (120g)	11	48	0.5
	Per 100g	9	40	0.4
Lemons, whole	1 large (120g)	4	22	0.4
	Per 100g	3.3	18	0.3
Lychees, canned in syrup	1 serving (160g)	30	112	tr
	Per 100g	19	70	tr
Lychees, raw	1 serving (120g)	17	66	0.1
	Per 100g	14	55	0.1
Lychees, raw weighed with skin and stones	1 serving (120g)	11	42	0.1
	Per 100g	9	35	0.1
Mandarin oranges, canned in syrup	1 serving (120g)	16	60	tr
	Per 100g	13	50	tr
Mandarin oranges, canned in juice	1 serving (120g)	10	40	tr
	Per 100g	8	33	tr
Mangoes canned in syrup	1 serving (160g)	32	128	tr
	Per 100g	20	80	tr

FOOD	SERVING	CARBS (g)	CALS (kcal)	FAT (g)
Mangoes, ripe, raw	1 whole (200g)	28	120	0.4
	Per 100g	14	60	0.2
Mangoes, with skin and stone	1 large (450g)	45	171	0.5
	Per 100g	10	38	0.1
Melon, Cantaloupe	1 serving (160g)	6	30	0.2
	Per 100g	3.9	19	0.1
Melon, Galia	1 serving (160g)	10	40	0.2
	Per 100g	6	25	0.1
Melon, Honeydew	1 serving (160g)	11	43	0.2
	Per 100g	7	27	0.1
Melon, watermelon	1 serving (160g)	11	48	0.5
	Per 100g	7	30	0.3
Mixed peel	1 serving (160g)	96	352	1.4
	Per 100g	60	220	0.9
Nectarines	1 average (120g)	11	48	0.1
	Per 100g	9	40	0.1
Olives, in brine	6 medium (50g)	tr	50	6
	Per 100g	tr	100	11
Oranges, peeled	1 medium (130g)	12	47	0.1
	Per 100g	9	36	0.1
Passion Fruit	1 serving (120g)	7	42	0.5
	Per 100g	6	35	0.4
Paw – paw, raw	1 whole (120g)	11	44	0.1
	Per 100g	9	37	0.1
Paw, paw, canned in juice	1 serving (120g)	22	78	tr
	Per 100g	18	65	tr
Peaches, canned in syrup	1 serving (160g)	21	88	tr
	Per 100g	13	55	tr
Peaches, canned in juice	1 serving (160g)	16	62	tr
	Per 100g	10	39	tr
Peaches, raw	1 whole (160g)	13	51	0.2
	Per 100g	8	32	0.1
Pears, canned in juice	1 serving (160g)	14	54	tr
	Per 100g	9	34	tr

Calorie, Fat & Carbohydrate Counter

FOOD	SERVING	CARBS (g)	CALS (kcal)	FAT (g)
Pears, canned in syrup	1 serving (160g)	19	80	tr
	Per 100g	12	50	tr
Pears, raw	1 average (180g)	18	70	0.2
	Per 100g	10	39	0.1
Pineapple, canned in juice	1 serving (160g)	19	72	tr
	Per 100g	12	45	tr
Pineapple, canned in syrup	1 serving (160g)	27	104	tr
	Per 100g	17	65	tr
Pineapple, raw, peeled	1 slice (120g)	12	48	0.2
	Per 100g	10	40	0.2
Plums, canned in syrup	1 serving (160g)	26	96	tr
	Per 100g	16	60	tr
Plums, raw	1 average (110g)	10	39	0.1
	Per 100g	9	35	0.1
Plums, stewed with sugar	1 serving (160g)	30	120	0.2
	Per 100g	19	75	0.1
Plums, stewed without sugar	1 serving (160g)	11	48	0.2
	Per 100g	7	30	0.1
Prunes, canned in juice	1 serving (160g)	34	128	0.3
	Per 100g	21	80	0.2
Prunes, canned in syrup	1 serving (160g)	38	144	0.3
	Per 100g	24	90	0.2
Prunes, ready to eat	1 serving (160g)	56	232	0.6
	Per 100g	35	145	0.4
Raisins	1 serving (70g)	49	189	0.3
	Per 100g	70	270	0.4
Raspberries, canned in syrup	1 serving (120g)	29	108	0.1
	Per 100g	24	90	0.1
Raspberries, raw	1 serving (60g)	3	16	0.2
	Per 100g	5	26	0.3
Rhubarb, canned in syrup	1 serving (160g)	13	51	tr
	Per 100g	8	32	tr
Rhubarb, raw	1 serving (120g)	1	8	0.1
	Per 100g	0.8	7	0.1

Fruit

FOOD	SERVING	CARBS (g)	CALS (kcal)	FAT (g)
Rhubarb, stewed with sugar	1 serving (160g)	18	80	0.2
	Per 100g	11	50	0.1
Rhubarb, stewed without sugar	1 serving (160g)	1.1	11	0.2
	Per 100g	0.7	7	0.1
Satsumas	1 average (120g)	11	44	0.1
	Per 100g	9	37	0.1
Strawberries, canned in syrup	1 serving (120g)	20	84	tr
	Per 100g	17	70	tr
Strawberries	1 serving (60g)	3.6	16	0.1
	Per 100g	6	27	0.1
Sultanas	1 serving (70g)	49	193	0.3
	Per 100g	70	275	0.4
Tangerines	1 average (120g)	7	30	0.1
	Per 100g	6	25	0.1

FOOD	SERVING	CARBS (g)	CALS (kcal)	FAT (g)

VEGETABLES

FOOD	SERVING	CARBS (g)	CALS (kcal)	FAT (g)
Aduki beans, cooked	1 serving (85g)	20	106	0.2
	Per 100g	23	125	0.2
Alfalfa sprouts, raw	1 serving (85g)	0.3	21	0.6
	Per 100g	0.4	25	0.7
Artichoke hearts, canned	1 heart (50g)	1	8	0
	Per 100g	1.9	16	0
Artichoke, Jerusalem, boiled	1 medium (100g)	10	40	0
	Per 100g	10	40	0
Artichoke, raw	1 medium (300g)	33	141	0.6
	Per 100g	11	47	0.2
Artichokes, globe, cooked, drained	1 medium (220g)	6	22	0.2
	Per 100g	2.6	10	0.1
Asparagus, canned, drained	5 spears (60g)	0.9	14	0.2
	Per 100g	1.5	23	0.3
Asparagus, fresh, boiled	5 spears (150g)	1.2	20	0
	Per 100g	0.8	13	0
Asparagus, raw	5 spears (160g)	3	40	1
	Per 100g	1.9	25	0.6
Aubergine, fried in corn oil	1 serving (120g)	3.5	378	38
	Per 100g	2.9	315	32
Aubergine, raw	1 small (120g)	2.5	18	0.5
	Per 100g	2.1	15	0.4
Avocado pear	1 medium (145g)	2.9	290	28
	Per 100g	2	200	19
Baked beans, canned in tomato sauce	1 serving (85g)	13	68	0.5
	Per 100g	15	80	0.6
Balor beans, canned	1 serving (85g)	2.3	16	0.1
	Per 100g	2.7	19	0.1
Bamboo shoots, canned	1 serving (140g)	1.7	13	0
	Per 100g	1.2	9	0
Bamboo shoots, raw	1 serving (120g)	7	32	0
	Per 100g	6	27	0

FOOD	SERVING	CARBS (g)	CALS (kcal)	FAT (g)
Bean sprouts, mung, cooked, drained	1 serving (85g)	0.7	9	0.1
	Per 100g	0.8	10	0.1
Bean sprouts, mung, raw	1 serving (85g)	3.4	26	0.4
	Per 100g	4	31	0.5
Beansprouts, raw	1 serving (85g)	3.4	29	0.4
	Per 100g	4	34	0.5
Beansprouts, stir fried	1 serving (85g)	2.1	64	5
	Per 100g	2.5	75	6
Beetroot, boiled	1 serving (85g)	9	38	0.1
	Per 100g	10	45	0.1
Beetroot, pickled, drained	4 slices (80g)	12	52	0
	Per 100g	15	65	0
Beetroot, raw	1 medium (120g)	8	42	0.1
	Per 100g	7	35	0.1
Black gram, cooked	1 serving (85g)	12	72	0.3
	Per 100g	14	85	0.4
Black kidney beans, cooked	1 serving (85g)	20	106	0.4
	Per 100g	24	125	0.5
Black-eyed beans, cooked	1 serving (85g)	18	98	0.6
	Per 100g	21	115	0.7
Borlotti beans, canned	1 serving (85g)	15	85	0.3
	Per 100g	18	100	0.4
Borlotti beans, cooked	1 serving (85g)	24	128	0.4
	Per 100g	28	150	0.5
Broad beans, fresh, cooked	1 serving (85g)	5	43	0.7
	Per 100g	6	50	0.8
Broad beans, raw	1 serving (85g)	6	51	0.9
	Per 100g	7	60	1
Broad beans,canned, reheated, drained	1 serving (85g)	11	72	0.6
	Per 100g	13	85	0.7
Broccoli, boiled in salted water	1 serving (80g)	0.9	19	0.6
	Per 100g	1.1	24	0.8
Broccoli, boiled in unsalted water	1 serving (80g)	0.9	20	0.6
	Per 100g	1.1	25	0.8

Calorie, Fat & Carbohydrate Counter

FOOD	SERVING	CARBS (g)	CALS (kcal)	FAT (g)
Broccoli, green, raw	1 serving (80g)	1.5	27	0.7
	Per 100g	1.9	34	0.9
Broccoli, purple sprouting boiled in salted water	1 serving (80g)	1.1	14	0.5
	Per 100g	1.4	18	0.6
Broccoli, purple sprouting boiled in unsalted water	1 serving (80g)	1	16	0.5
	Per 100g	1.3	20	0.6
Broccoli, purple sprouting, raw	1 serving (80g)	1.5	29	0.6
	Per 100g	1.9	36	0.7
Brussels sprouts, boiled in salted water	1 serving (80g)	2.9	28	1.1
	Per 100g	3.6	35	1.4
Brussels sprouts, boiled in unsalted water	1 serving (80g)	2.9	29	1
	Per 100g	3.6	36	1.3
Brussels sprouts, canned, drained	1 serving (80g)	2	22	0.8
	Per 100g	2.5	28	1
Brussels sprouts, raw	1 serving (80g)	2.3	27	0.4
	Per 100g	2.9	34	0.5
Butter beans, boiled	1 serving (85g)	15	94	0.5
	Per 100g	18	110	0.6
Butter beans, canned, drained	1 serving (85g)	12	64	0.4
	Per 100g	14	75	0.5
Butter beans, raw	1 serving (85g)	47	247	1.5
	Per 100g	55	290	1.8
Cabbage, boiled	1 serving (80g)	1.8	13	0.3
	Per 100g	2.3	16	0.4
Cabbage, chinese, pak-choi, raw	1 serving (60g)	0	8	0
	Per 100g	0	13	0
Cabbage, Chinese, raw	1 serving (60g)	0.6	3.6	0.1
	Per 100g	1	6	0.2
Cabbage, raw	1 serving (60g)	2.3	15	0.2
	Per 100g	3.9	25	0.4
Cabbage, red, boiled	1 serving (80g)	1.8	11	0.2
	Per 100g	2.3	14	0.3
Cabbage, red, raw	1 serving (60g)	2.2	13	0.2
	Per 100g	3.7	22	0.3

FOOD	SERVING	CARBS (g)	CALS (kcal)	FAT (g)
Cabbage, Savoy, cooked	1 serving (60g)	1	10	0.1
	Per 100g	1.7	17	0.2
Cabbage, Savoy, raw	1 serving (60g)	2.3	16	0.3
	Per 100g	3.9	27	0.5
Cabbage, white, boiled	1 serving (60g)	1.3	8	0.1
	Per 100g	2.1	14	0.2
Cabbage, white, raw	1 serving (60g)	3	16	0.1
	Per 100g	5	26	0.2
Cannellini beans, canned	1 serving (85g)	11	72	0.4
	Per 100g	13	85	0.5
Carrot juice	1 small glass (125ml)	8	0	39
	Per 100ml	6	33	0.1
Carrots, baby, boiled	1 serving (85g)	3.4	15	0.3
	Per 100g	4	18	0.4
Carrots, baby, raw	1 serving (85g)	5	24	0.3
	Per 100g	6	28	0.4
Carrots, canned, drained	1 serving (85g)	3.4	18	0.2
	Per 100g	4	21	0.2
Carrots, frozen	1 serving (85g)	4	22	0.3
	Per 100g	5	26	0.4
Carrots, raw	1 medium (120g)	7	29	0.2
	Per 100g	6	24	0.2
Carrots, whole, boiled	1 serving (85g)	5	25	0.1
	Per 100g	6	29	0.1
Cauliflower, boiled	1 serving (80g)	1.7	22	0.7
	Per 100g	2.1	27	0.9
Cauliflower, raw	1 serving (80g)	2.4	26	0.7
	Per 100g	3	33	0.9
Celeriac, boiled	1 serving (80g)	1.5	12	0.4
	Per 100g	1.9	15	0.5
Celeriac, raw	1 serving (80g)	1.9	14	0.3
	Per 100g	2.4	18	0.4
Celery, boiled	1 serving (60g)	1.6	8	0.1
	Per 100g	2.6	13	0.2

Calorie, Fat & Carbohydrate Counter

FOOD	SERVING	CARBS (g)	CALS (kcal)	FAT (g)
Celery, raw	1 med stalk (40g)	0.4	2.8	0.1
	Per 100g	1	7	0.2
Chickpeas, canned, drained	1 serving (60g)	10	69	1.8
	Per 100g	16	115	3
Chickpeas, split, dried, boiled	1 serving (60g)	11	72	1.2
	Per 100g	18	120	2
Chickpeas, split, dried, raw	1 serving (60g)	30	189	3
	Per 100g	50	315	5
Chickpeas, whole, dried, boiled	1 serving (60g)	10	69	1.3
	Per 100g	17	115	2.2
Chickpeas, whole, dried, raw	1 serving (60g)	30	195	3
	Per 100g	50	325	5
Chicory, raw	1 serving (60g)	1.7	7	0.4
	Per 100g	2.9	11	0.6
Chives	fresh, 2 tbsp (40g)	0.6	8	0.2
	Per 100g	1.5	19	0.6
Courgette, boiled in unsalted water	1 serving (60g)	1.1	11	0.2
	Per 100g	1.9	19	0.4
Courgette, fried in corn oil	1 serving (60g)	1.6	39	3
	Per 100g	2.7	65	5
Courgette, raw	1 serving (60g)	1.1	10	0.2
	Per 100g	1.8	17	0.4
Cucumber	5 average slices (80g)	1.2	8	0.1
	Per 100g	1.5	10	0.1
Curly kale, boiled in unsalted water	1 serving (60g)	0.6	14	0.7
	Per 100g	1	23	1.1
Curly kale, raw	1 serving (60g)	0.8	19	1
	Per 100g	1.4	32	1.7
Fennel, boiled in salted water	1 bulb (150g)	2.3	17	0.3
	Per 100g	1.5	11	0.2
Fennel, raw	1 bulb (150g)	2.7	18	0.3
	Per 100g	1.8	12	0.2
Garlic, raw	2 peeled cloves (6g)	1	6	0
	Per 100g	16	95	0.6

FOOD	SERVING	CARBS (g)	CALS (kcal)	FAT (g)
Gherkins, pickled and drained	1 serving (60g)	1.6	8	0.1
	Per 100g	2.7	14	0.1
Gourd, raw	1 serving (60g)	0.5	7	0.1
	Per 100g	0.8	11	0.2
Green beans, French beans, canned	1 serving (85g)	3.4	19	0.1
	Per 100g	4	22	0.1
Green beans, French beans, raw	1 serving (85g)	2.7	20	0.4
	Per 100g	3.2	23	0.5
Green beans, fresh, cooked	1 serving (85g)	2.5	18	0
	Per 100g	2.9	21	0
Green beans, frozen, cooked	1 serving (85g)	4	20	0
	Per 100g	5	24	0
Haricot beans, cooked	1 serving (85g)	14	77	0.4
	Per 100g	17	90	0.5
Kidney beans, red, canned, drained, heated	1 serving (85g)	9	60	0.4
	Per 100g	11	70	0.5
Leeks, boiled in unsalted water	1 serving (60g)	1.5	13	0.4
	Per 100g	2.5	21	0.7
Leeks, raw	1 serving (60g)	1.7	13	0.3
	Per 100g	2.9	22	0.5
Lentils, canned in tomato sauce	1 serving (60g)	5	33	0.1
	Per 100g	9	55	0.2
Lentils, Green & Brown, whole, dried, cooked	1 serving (60g)	10	63	0.4
	Per 100g	17	105	0.7
Lentils, Green & Brown, whole, dried, raw	1 serving (60g)	30	183	1.1
	Per 100g	50	305	1.9
Lentils, red, split, cooked	1 serving (60g)	11	60	0.2
	Per 100g	18	100	0.4
Lentils, red, split, raw	1 serving (60g)	33	183	0.8
	Per 100g	55	305	1.3
Lentils, whole, dried, cooked	1 serving (60g)	10	66	0.4
	Per 100g	17	110	0.6
Lettuce, butterhead	1 serving (40g)	0.5	5	0.2
	Per 100g	1.2	12	0.6

Calorie, Fat & Carbohydrate Counter

FOOD	SERVING	CARBS (g)	CALS (kcal)	FAT (g)
Lettuce, iceberg	1 serving (40g)	0.8	5	0.1
	Per 100g	1.9	12	0.3
Lettuce, raw	1 serving (40g)	0.6	6	0.2
	Per 100g	1.6	15	0.5
Lima beans, dried, cooked	1 tbsp (about 30g)	3	21	tr
	Per 100g	10	70	tr
Marrow, boiled in unsalted water	1 serving (85g)	1.4	8	0.2
	Per 100g	1.6	9	0.2
Marrow, raw	1 serving (85g)	1.9	10	0.2
	Per 100g	2.2	12	0.2
Mixed vegetables, frozen, boiled	1 serving (85g)	6	38	0.4
	Per 100g	7	45	0.5
Mung beans, cooked	1 serving (60g)	9	54	0.2
	Per 100g	15	90	0.4
Mung beans, Dahl, dried, cooked	1 serving (60g)	9	54	0.2
	Per 100g	15	90	0.4
Mung beans, Dahl, dried, raw	1 serving (60g)	27	174	0.6
	Per 100g	45	290	1
Mung beans, whole, dried, raw	1 serving (60g)	27	174	0.6
	Per 100g	45	290	1
Mushrooms, boiled in salted water	1 serving (60g)	0.2	7	0.2
	Per 100g	0.4	11	0.3
Mushrooms, common, raw	1 serving (60g)	0.2	8	0.3
	Per 100g	0.4	13	0.5
Mushrooms, fried in corn oil	1 serving (60g)	0.2	96	10
	Per 100g	0.3	160	16
Mustard and cress, raw	1 serving (60g)	0.2	8	0.4
	Per 100g	0.4	13	0.6
Okra, boiled in unsalted water	1 serving (60g)	1.7	17	0.5
	Per 100g	2.8	29	0.9
Okra, raw	1 serving (60g)	1.7	18	0.6
	Per 100g	2.9	30	1
Okra, stir fried in corn oil	1 serving (60g)	2.3	159	16
	Per 100g	3.9	265	27

FOOD	SERVING	CARBS (g)	CALS (kcal)	FAT (g)
Onions, boiled in unsalted water	1 serving (60g)	2.2	10	0.1
	Per 100g	3.7	16	0.1
Onions, cocktail / silverskin, drained	1 serving (60g)	1.9	9	0.1
	Per 100g	3.1	15	0.1
Onions, fried in blended oil	1 serving (60g)	8	102	7
	Per 100g	14	170	11
Onions, fried in corn oil	1 serving (60g)	8	102	7
	Per 100g	14	170	12
Onions, fried in lard	1 serving (60g)	9	99	7
	Per 100g	15	165	11
Onions, pickled and drained	1 serving (60g)	3	14	0.1
	Per 100g	5	23	0.2
Onions, raw	1 serving (60g)	5	21	0.1
	Per 100g	8	35	0.2
Parsnip, boiled in unsalted water	1 serving (85g)	10	55	1
	Per 100g	12	65	1.2
Parsnip, raw	1 average (160g)	21	104	1.8
	Per 100g	13	65	1.1
Peppers, capsicum, chilli, green, raw	1 average (20g)	0.1	4	0.1
	Per 100g	0.7	20	0.6
Peppers, capsicum, green, raw	1 serving (85g)	2.2	13	0.3
	Per 100g	2.6	15	0.3
Peppers, capsicum, red, raw	1 serving (85g)	5	26	0.3
	Per 100g	6	31	0.4
Peppers, green boiled in salted water	1 serving (85g)	2.2	15	0.4
	Per 100g	2.6	18	0.5
Peppers, red boiled in salted water	1 serving (85g)	6	28	0.3
	Per 100g	7	33	0.4
Pinto beans, dried, boiled	1 serving (85g)	21	115	0.6
	Per 100g	25	135	0.7
Pinto beans, dried, raw	1 serving (85g)	47	281	1.4
	Per 100g	55	330	1.6
Pinto beans, refried	1 serving (85g)	13	89	0.9
	Per 100g	15	105	1.1

Calorie, Fat & Carbohydrate Counter

FOOD	SERVING	CARBS (g)	CALS (kcal)	FAT (g)
Plantain, boiled in unsalted water	1 serving (60g)	17	72	0.1
	Per 100g	28	120	0.2
Plantain, raw	1 serving (60g)	18	69	0.2
	Per 100g	30	115	0.3
Plantain, ripe, fried in oil	1 serving (60g)	30	165	5
	Per 100g	50	275	9
Potato, baked, jacket	1 serving (150g)	21	113	1.1
	Per 100g	14	75	0.7
Potato, boiled, peeled	1 serving (150g)	20	98	0.5
	Per 100g	13	65	0.3
Potato, boiled, unpeeled	1 serving (150g)	20	98	0
	Per 100g	13	65	0
Potato, chips, oven cook	1 serving (100g)	26	130	3
	Per 100g	26	130	3
Potato, hash brown	1 serving (55g)	14	176	12
	Per 100g	26	320	22
Potato, new, peeled	1 serving (165g)	20	99	0
	Per 100g	12	60	0
Potato, oven fried	1 serving (100g)	30	240	13
	Per 100g	30	240	13
Potato, roast, no skin	1 serving (150g)	27	165	4
	Per 100g	18	110	2.8
Potato, roast, with skin	1 serving (150g)	24	165	4
	Per 100g	16	110	2.6
Potato, steamed, new, peeled	1 serving (165g)	20	99	0
	Per 100g	12	60	0
Potato, wedges, crunchy	1 serving (100g)	26	170	6
	Per 100g	26	170	6
Potato,fried, thin cut	1 serving (150g)	45	330	18
	Per 100g	30	220	12
Pumpkin, boiled in salted water	1 serving (85g)	1.8	12	0.3
	Per 100g	2.1	14	0.3
Pumpkin, raw	1 serving (85g)	1.9	12	0.2
	Per 100g	2.2	14	0.2

FOOD	SERVING	CARBS (g)	CALS (kcal)	FAT (g)
Quorn	1 serving (60g)	1.1	54	2
	Per 100g	1.9	90	3.3
Radish, raw	4 average (60g)	1.1	7	0.1
	Per 100g	1.8	12	0.2
Runner beans, fresh, cooked	1 serving (85g)	2	14	0.4
	Per 100g	2.4	17	0.5
Runner beans, raw	1 serving (85g)	2.8	18	0.3
	Per 100g	3.3	21	0.4
Soya beans, canned in tomato sauce	1 serving (85g)	6	77	2.6
	Per 100g	7	90	3
Soya beans, canned, drained, cooked	1 serving (85g)	4	119	6
	Per 100g	5	140	7
Soya beans, dried, cooked	1 serving (85g)	1.3	106	7
	Per 100g	1.5	125	8
Soya beans, dried, raw	1 serving (85g)	14	310	15
	Per 100g	17	365	18
Spinach, boiled in unsalted water	1 serving (60g)	0.5	12	0.5
	Per 100g	0.8	20	0.8
Spinach, frozen, boiled in unsalted water	1 serving (60g)	0.3	13	0.5
	Per 100g	0.5	21	0.8
Spinach, raw	1 serving (60g)	1	16	0.5
	Per 100g	1.6	26	0.8
Spring greens, boiled in unsalted water	1 serving (60g)	1	12	0.4
	Per 100g	1.7	20	0.7
Spring greens, raw	1 serving (60g)	1.8	19	0.6
	Per 100g	3	32	1
Spring onions, raw	1 serving (60g)	1.9	13	0.3
	Per 100g	3.1	22	0.5
Swede, boiled in unsalted water	1 serving (85g)	1.9	9	0.1
	Per 100g	2.2	11	0.1
Swede, raw	1 serving (85g)	4	21	0.3
	Per 100g	5	25	0.3
Sweet potato, boiled in salted water	1 serving (85g)	18	72	0.3
	Per 100g	21	85	0.3

Calorie, Fat & Carbohydrate Counter

FOOD	SERVING	CARBS (g)	CALS (kcal)	FAT (g)
Sweet potato, raw	1 potato (200g)	42	170	0.6
	Per 100g	21	85	0.3
Sweetcorn, baby, canned	1 serving (60g)	1.2	14	0.2
	Per 100g	2	23	0.4
Sweetcorn, kernels, canned	1 serving (60g)	17	72	0.7
	Per 100g	28	120	1.2
Sweetcorn, on-the-cob, boiled	1 serving (60g)	7	39	0.8
	Per 100g	12	65	1.4
Tomato puree	1 serving (60g)	8	42	0.1
	Per 100g	13	70	0.2
Tomatoes, canned, whole	1 serving (85g)	2.5	14	0.1
	Per 100g	2.9	16	0.1
Tomatoes, fried in blended oil	1 serving (85g)	4	81	7
	Per 100g	5	95	8
Tomatoes, fried in corn oil	1 serving (85g)	4	81	7
	Per 100g	5	95	8
Tomatoes, fried in lard	1 serving (85g)	4	72	7
	Per 100g	5	85	8
Tomatoes, grilled	1 serving (85g)	8	43	0.8
	Per 100g	9	50	0.9
Tomatoes, raw	1 tomato (120g)	3.7	20	0.4
	Per 100g	3.1	17	0.3
Turnip, boiled in unsalted water	1 serving (85g)	1.8	11	0.2
	Per 100g	2.1	13	0.2
Turnip, raw	1 serving (85g)	4	20	0.3
	Per 100g	5	23	0.3
Watercress, raw	1 serving (60g)	0.2	14	0.6
	Per 100g	0.4	23	1
Yam, boiled in unsalted water	1 serving (85g)	30	115	0.3
	Per 100g	35	135	0.3
Yam, raw	1 serving (85g)	25	98	0.3
	Per 100g	29	115	0.3

FOOD	SERVING	CARBS (g)	CALS (kcal)	FAT (g)
HERBS AND SPICES				
Basil, dried, ground	1 tsp (2g)	0.9	5.0	0.1
	Per 100g	43	251	4
Basil, fresh	1 tbsp (5g)	0.3	2.0	0
	Per 100g	5.1	40	0.8
Chilli powder	1 tsp (2g)	0	0	0.3
	Per 100g	0	0	17
Cinnamon, ground	1 tsp (2g)	0	0	0.1
	Per 100g	0	0	3.1
Coriander, dried	1 tsp (2g)	0.8	5.6	0.1
	Per 100g	40	280	4.5
Coriander, fresh	1 tbsp (5g)	0.1	1.3	0
	Per 100g	2.1	25	0.7
Curry powder	1 tsp (2g)	0.5	4.8	0.2
	Per 100g	26	240	11
Mint, fresh	1 tbsp (5g)	0.3	2	0
	Per 100g	5	40	0.7
Mustard powder	1 tsp (2g)	0.4	9.3	0.6
	Per 100g	21	465	30
Paprika	1 tsp (2g)	0.7	5.7	0.3
	Per 100g	35	285	13
Parsley, fresh	1 tbsp (5g)	0.1	1.7	0.1
	Per 100g	2.7	33	1.3
Pepper, black	1 tsp (2g)	0	0	0.1
	Per 100g	0	0	3.2
Pepper, white	1 tsp (2g)	0	0	0
	Per 100g	0	0	2.2
Rosemary, dried	1 tbsp (5g)	2.3	16	0.8
	Per 100g	45	315	16
Sage, dried, ground	1 tbsp (5g)	2.3	16	0.7
	Per 100g	45	315	13
Thyme, dried, ground	1 tbsp (5g)	2.3	14	0.4
	Per 100g	45	285	7

Calorie, Fat & Carbohydrate Counter

FOOD	SERVING	CARBS (g)	CALS (kcal)	FAT (g)

FISH

Seafood

FOOD	SERVING	CARBS (g)	CALS (kcal)	FAT (g)
Anchovies, canned in oil, drained	1 anchovy (5g)	0	14	1
	Per 100g	0	270	20
Bass, sea, mixed species	1 serving (130g)	0	150	3.3
	Per 100g	0	115	2.5
Bass, striped	1 serving (130g)	0	117	3.3
	Per 100g	0	90	2.5
Bluefish	1 serving (130g)	0	150	5
	Per 100g	0	115	4
Carp	1 serving (130g)	0	215	9
	Per 100g	0	165	7
Catfish, channel, uncooked	1 serving (130g)	0	150	5
	Per 100g	0	115	3.8
Catfish, channel, breaded and fried	1 serving (130g)	10	299	17
	Per 100g	8	230	13
Caviar, black or red	1 Tbsp (16g)	0.5	38	3
	Per 100g	3.1	240	19
Cod fillets, poached	1 serving (130g)	0	124	1.4
	Per 100g	0	95	1.1
Cod fillets, poached, weighed with skin	1 serving (130g)	0	104	1.3
	Per 100g	0	80	1
Cod, baked, fillets	1 serving (130g)	0	124	1.6
	Per 100g	0	95	1.2
Cod, dried, salted, boiled	1 serving (130g)	0	182	1.2
	Per 100g	0	140	0.9
Cod, fillets, weighed with skin	1 serving (130g)	0	111	1.3
	Per 100g	0	85	1
Cod, grilled, steaks	1 serving (130g)	0	130	1.7
	Per 100g	0	100	1.3
Cod, in batter, fried in dripping	1 serving (130g)	10	260	13
	Per 100g	8	200	10

FOOD	SERVING	CARBS (g)	CALS (kcal)	FAT (g)
Cod, in batter, fried in oil	1 serving (130g)	10	267	13
	Per 100g	8	205	10
Cod, raw, fillets	1 serving (130g)	0	98	0.9
	Per 100g	0	75	0.7
Croaker, Atlantic, breaded and fried	1 serving (130g)	10	280	18
	Per 100g	8	215	14
Croaker, Atlantic, uncooked	1 serving (130g)	0	137	4
	Per 100g	0	105	3.1
Dogfish, in batter, fried in dripping	1 serving (130g)	10	338	26
	Per 100g	8	260	20
Dogfish, in batter, fried in oil	1 serving (130g)	10	345	23
	Per 100g	8	265	18
Eel	1 serving (130g)	0	306	20
	Per 100g	0	235	15
Flounder	1 serving (130g)	0	143	2
	Per 100g	0	110	1.5
Grouper	1 serving (130g)	0	156	1.7
	Per 100g	0	120	1.3
Haddock, in crumbs, fried in dripping, with bones and skin	1 serving (130g)	4	215	10
	Per 100g	3.2	165	8
Haddock, in crumbs, fried in oil	1 serving (130g)	5	234	10
	Per 100g	3.7	180	8
Haddock, in crumbs, fried in oil, with bones and skin	1 serving (130g)	4	208	10
	Per 100g	3.3	160	8
Haddock, in crumbs, fried with dripping	1 serving (130g)	5	228	10
	Per 100g	3.7	175	8
Haddock, raw	1 serving (130g)	0	91	0.8
	Per 100g	0	70	0.6
Haddock, smoked, steamed	1 serving (130g)	0	130	1.2
	Per 100g	0	100	0.9

Calorie, Fat & Carbohydrate Counter

FOOD	SERVING	CARBS (g)	CALS (kcal)	FAT (g)
Haddock, smoked, steamed, with bones and skin	1 serving (130g)	0	91	0.8
	Per 100g	0	70	0.6
Haddock, steamed	1 serving (130g)	0	124	1
	Per 100g	0	95	0.8
Haddock, steamed weighed with bones and skin	1 serving (130g)	0	98	0.8
	Per 100g	0	75	0.6
Halibut, raw	1 serving (130g)	0	124	3
	Per 100g	0	95	2.3
Halibut, steamed	1 serving (130g)	0	163	5
	Per 100g	0	125	4
Halibut, steamed, weighed with bones and skin	1 serving (130g)	0	130	4
	Per 100g	0	100	3.1
Herring, raw	1 serving (130g)	0	293	25
	Per 100g	0	225	19
Herring, fried	1 serving (130g)	2	319	20
	Per 100g	1.5	245	15
Herring, fried, weighed with bones	1 serving (130g)	1.7	260	17
	Per 100g	1.3	200	13
Herring, grilled	1 serving (130g)	0	260	17
	Per 100g	0	200	13
Herring, grilled, weighed with bones	1 serving (130g)	0	176	12
	Per 100g	0	135	9
Kipper, baked	1 serving (130g)	0	260	14
	Per 100g	0	200	11
Kipper, baked, weighed with bones	1 serving (130g)	0	143	8
	Per 100g	0	110	6
Lemon sole, in crumbs, fried	1 serving (130g)	12	293	16
	Per 100g	9	225	12
Lemon sole, in crumbs, fried, weighed with bones and skin	1 serving (130g)	9	215	13
	Per 100g	7	165	10

FOOD	SERVING	CARBS (g)	CALS (kcal)	FAT (g)
Lemon sole, raw	1 serving (130g)	0	104	2
	Per 100g	0	80	1.5
Lemon sole, steamed	1 serving (130g)	0	124	1.2
	Per 100g	0	95	0.9
Lemon sole, steamed weighed with skin and bones	1 serving (130g)	0	85	0.8
	Per 100g	0	65	0.6
Mackerel, Atlantic	1 serving (130g)	0	345	22
	Per 100g	0	265	17
Mackerel, king	1 serving (130g)	0	137	2.6
	Per 100g	0	105	2
Mackerel, Spanish	1 serving (130g)	0	208	8
	Per 100g	0	160	6
Mackerel, fried	1 serving (130g)	0	254	16
	Per 100g	0	195	12
Mackerel, fried, weighed with bones	1 serving (130g)	0	182	10
	Per 100g	0	140	8
Mackerel, raw	1 serving (130g)	0	280	21
	Per 100g	0	215	16
Mackerel, smoked	1 serving (130g)	0	468	39
	Per 100g	0	360	30
Mahi-mahi	1 serving (130g)	0	104	0.9
	Per 100g	0	80	0.7
Monkfish	1 serving (130g)	0	98	2.1
	Per 100g	0	75	1.6
Mullet, striped	1 serving (130g)	0	202	7
	Per 100g	0	155	5
Ocean perch, Atlantic	1 serving (130g)	0	150	2.7
	Per 100g	0	115	2.1
Octopus, common	1 serving (130g)	2.7	111	1.4
	Per 100g	2.1	85	1.1
Orange roughy	1 serving (130g)	0	85	0.9
	Per 100g	0	65	0.7

Calorie, Fat & Carbohydrate Counter

FOOD	SERVING	CARBS (g)	CALS (kcal)	FAT (g)
Pike, Northern	1 serving (130g)	0	150	1.2
	Per 100g	0	115	0.9
Pilchards, canned in tomato sauce	1 serving (130g)	0.9	163	7
	Per 100g	0.7	125	5
Plaice, in batter, fried in blended oil	1 serving (130g)	18	351	22
	Per 100g	14	270	17
Plaice, in batter, fried in dripping	1 serving (130g)	18	377	23
	Per 100g	14	290	18
Plaice, in crumbs, fried, fillets	1 serving (130g)	12	293	18
	Per 100g	9	225	14
Plaice, raw	1 serving (130g)	0	124	2.7
	Per 100g	0	95	2.1
Plaice, steamed	1 serving (130g)	0	117	2.6
	Per 100g	0	90	2
Plaice, steamed, weighed with bones	1 serving (130g)	0	65	1.3
	Per 100g	0	50	1
Pollack	1 serving (130g)	0	156	1.6
	Per 100g	0	120	1.2
Pompano, Florida	1 serving (130g)	0	280	16
	Per 100g	0	215	12
Roe, mixed species	1 serving (130g)	2	182	8
	Per 100g	1.5	140	6
Sablefish	1 serving (130g)	0	325	25
	Per 100g	0	250	19
Saithe, raw	1 serving (130g)	0	91	0.4
	Per 100g	0	70	0.3
Saithe, steamed	1 serving (130g)	0	130	0.8
	Per 100g	0	100	0.6
Saithe, steamed, weighed with bone and skin	1 serving (130g)	0	104	0.7
	Per 100g	0	80	0.5
Salmon, canned	1 serving (130g)	0	195	10
	Per 100g	0	150	8

FOOD	SERVING	CARBS (g)	CALS (kcal)	FAT (g)
Salmon, Chinook	1 serving (130g)	0	150	5
	Per 100g	0	115	4
Salmon, chum, canned	1 serving (130g)	0	182	8
	Per 100g	0	140	6
Salmon, coho	1 serving (130g)	0	241	10
	Per 100g	0	185	8
Salmon, pink, canned, with bones & liquid	1 serving (130g)	0	182	8
	Per 100g	0	140	6
Salmon, raw	1 serving (130g)	0	234	14
	Per 100g	0	180	11
Salmon, smoked	1 serving (130g)	0	189	7
	Per 100g	0	145	5
Salmon, sockeye, canned, with bones	1 serving (130g)	0	195	9
	Per 100g	0	150	7
Salmon, sockeye, fresh	1 serving (130g)	0	280	14
	Per 100g	0	215	11
Salmon, steamed	1 serving (130g)	0	267	17
	Per 100g	0	205	13
Salmon, steamed, weighed with bone	1 serving (130g)	0	208	14
	Per 100g	0	160	11
Sardines, Atlantic, canned in oil	2 (about 30g)	0	50	2.8
	Per 100g	0	175	10
Sardines, canned in oil	1 serving (130g)	0	293	18
	Per 100g	0	225	14
Sardines, canned in tomato sauce	1 serving (130g)	0.7	241	17
	Per 100g	0.5	185	13
Shad, American	1 serving (130g)	0	267	18
	Per 100g	0	205	14
Shark, mixed species	1 serving (130g)	0	163	5
	Per 100g	0	125	3.9
Skate, in batter, fried	1 serving (130g)	7	260	16
	Per 100g	5	200	12
Smelt, rainbow	1 serving (130g)	0	163	4
	Per 100g	0	125	3

Calorie, Fat & Carbohydrate Counter

FOOD	SERVING	CARBS (g)	CALS (kcal)	FAT (g)
Snapper, mixed species	1 serving (130g)	0	163	2.3
	Per 100g	0	125	1.8
Sole	1 serving (130g)	0	150	2
	Per 100g	0	115	1.5
Squid, mixed species	1 serving (130g)	10	221	10
	Per 100g	8	170	8
Sturgeon, mixed species	1 serving (130g)	0	234	5
	Per 100g	0	180	4
Surimi	1 serving (130g)	9	124	1
	Per 100g	7	95	0.8
Swordfish, cooked dry heat	1 serving (130g)	0	195	7
	Per 100g	0	150	5
Tilefish, cooked dry heat	1 serving (130g)	0	189	7
	Per 100g	0	145	5
Trout, brown, steamed	1 serving (130g)	0	169	7
	Per 100g	0	130	5
Trout, rainbow, cooked dry heat	1 serving (130g)	0	195	5
	Per 100g	0	150	4
Trout, steamed, weighed with bones	1 serving (130g)	0	117	3.8
	Per 100g	0	90	2.9
Tuna, canned in brine, drained	1 serving (130g)	0	130	0.8
	Per 100g	0	100	0.6
Tuna, canned in oil, drained	1 serving (130g)	0	247	12
	Per 100g	0	190	9
Tuna, fresh	1 serving (130g)	0	234	8
	Per 100g	0	180	6
Tuna, light meat, canned in water	1 serving (130g)	0	176	0.7
	Per 100g	0	135	0.5
Tuna, white, canned in water	1 serving (130g)	0	169	3.3
	Per 100g	0	130	2.5
Turbot, European	1 serving (130g)	0	130	3.9
	Per 100g	0	100	3
Whitebait, fried	1 serving (130g)	7	696	65
	Per 100g	5	535	50

FOOD	SERVING	CARBS (g)	CALS (kcal)	FAT (g)
Whitefish, mixed species, cooked in dry heat	1 serving (130g)	0	137	1.2
	Per 100g	0	105	0.9
Whiting, in crumbs, fried	1 serving (130g)	9	260	13
	Per 100g	7	200	10
Whiting, in crumbs, fried, weighed with bones	1 serving (130g)	8	221	12
	Per 100g	6	170	9
Whiting, steamed	1 serving (130g)	0	124	1.2
	Per 100g	0	95	0.9
Whiting, steamed, weighed with bone and skin	1 serving (130g)	0	85	0.8
	Per 100g	0	65	0.6

Shellfish

FOOD	SERVING	CARBS (g)	CALS (kcal)	FAT (g)
Abalone, fried	1 serving (90g)	10	171	6
	Per 100g	11	190	7
Clams, mixed species, canned	1 serving (90g)	5	131	1.8
	Per 100g	5	145	2
Clams, mixed species, steamed	20 small (about 85g)	4	133	1.8
	Per 100g	5	160	2
Cockles, boiled	1 serving (130g)	tr	65	0.4
	Per 100g	tr	50	0.3
Crab, Alaskan king, steamed	1 serving (130g)	0	124	2
	Per 100g	0	95	1.5
Crab, blue, cooked	1 serving (130g)	0	130	2.2
	Per 100g	0	100	1.7
Crab, boiled	1 serving (130g)	0	156	7
	Per 100g	0	120	5
Crab, boiled, weighed with shell	1 serving (130g)	0	33	1.3
	Per 100g	0	25	1
Crab, canned	1 serving (130g)	0	104	1.2
	Per 100g	0	80	0.9
Crab, soft-shell, fried	1 serving (130g)	33	345	18
	Per 100g	25	265	14
Crayfish, steamed	1 serving (90g)	0	99	1.2
	Per 100g	0	110	1.3

Calorie, Fat & Carbohydrate Counter

FOOD	SERVING	CARBS (g)	CALS (kcal)	FAT (g)
Lobster, steamed	1 serving (130g)	1.7	124	0.8
	Per 100g	1.3	95	0.6
Lobster, boiled	1 serving (130g)	0	163	4
	Per 100g	0	125	3
Lobster, boiled, weighed with shell	1 serving (130g)	0	59	1.6
	Per 100g	0	45	1
Mussels, blue, cooked	1 serving (130g)	9	228	5
	Per 100g	7	175	4
Mussels, boiled	1 serving (130g)	tr	117	2.6
	Per 100g	tr	90	2
Mussels, boiled, weighed with shell	1 serving (130g)	tr	35	0.8
	Per 100g	tr	27	0.6
Oysters, raw	10 average (60g)	0.5	69	2.3
	Per 100g	0.8	115	3.9
Oysters, smoked, canned in oil, drained	10 average (60g)	0.5	129	7
	Per 100g	0.8	215	12
Prawns, boiled	1 serving (130g)	0	143	2.5
	Per 100g	0	110	1.9
Prawns, boiled, weighed with shell	1 serving (130g)	0	52	0.9
	Per 100g	0	40	0.7
Scallops, mixed species, breaded and fried	2 large (about 30g)	3.3	71	1
	Per 100g	11	225	3.4
Scampi, in breadcrumbs, frozen, fried	1 serving (130g)	26	383	20
	Per 100g	20	295	15
Shrimp, mixed species, fried	1 serving (90g)	0	212	11
	Per 100g	0	235	12
Shrimp, mixed species, steamed	1 serving (90g)	0	90	1
	Per 100g	0	100	1.1
Shrimps, canned, drained	1 serving (130g)	0	124	1.7
	Per 100g	0	95	1.3
Shrimps, frozen, shell removed	1 serving (130g)	0	98	1
	Per 100g	0	75	0.8
Squid, frozen, raw	1 serving (130g)	0	91	2
	Per 100g	0	70	1.5

FOOD	SERVING	CARBS (g)	CALS (kcal)	FAT (g)
Whelks, boiled, weighed with shell	1 serving (130g)	tr	20	0.4
	Per 100g	tr	15	0.3

Fish products

FOOD	SERVING	CARBS (g)	CALS (kcal)	FAT (g)
Fish cakes, fried	1 fish cake (50g)	8	90	6
	Per 100g	16	180	11
Fish fingers, fried in blended oil	1 fish finger (28g)	5	67	3.6
	Per 100g	17	240	13
Fish fingers, fried in lard	1 fish finger (28g)	5	64	3.6
	Per 100g	17	230	13
Fish fingers, grilled	1 fish finger (28g)	6	57	2.5
	Per 100g	20	205	9
Fish paste	1 thin spread (10g)	0.4	16	1
	Per 100g	3.6	160	10
Fish pie	1 serving (250g)	28	263	8
	Per 100g	11	105	3.1
Kedgeree	1 serving (250g)	28	413	20
	Per 100g	11	165	8
Roe, cod, hard, fried	1 serving (250g)	7	500	30
	Per 100g	2.9	200	12
Roe, herring, soft, fried	1 serving (250g)	13	613	40
	Per 100g	5	245	16
Taramasalata	1 serving (50g)	2	223	25
	Per 100g	3.9	445	50
Fisherman's pie	1 pie (300g)	27	360	15
	Per 100g	9	120	5
Fish lasagne	1 serving (250g)	33	363	18
	Per 100g	13	145	7
Fish curry	1 serving (250g)	3.8	313	20
	Per 100g	1.5	125	8

FOOD	SERVING	CARBS (g)	CALS (kcal)	FAT (g)

FATS, OILS, SAUCES AND NUTS

Fats

FOOD	SERVING	CARBS (g)	CALS (kcal)	FAT (g)
Butter	1 serving (10g)	0	7.5	8
	Per 100g	0.1	750	80
Butter, half fat	1 serving (10g)	0	36	4
	Per 100g	0.1	363	40
Compound cooking fat (suet)	1 serving (10g)	1	84	9
	Per 100g	12	835	85
Dripping (beef)	1 serving (10g)	0	87	9
	Per 100g	0	865	91
Gold, low fat spread	1 serving (10g)	0.3	27	2
	Per 100g	3	370	38
Lard	1 serving (10g)	0	92	10
	Per 100g	0	915	102
Low fat spread	1 serving (10g)	0	19	4
	Per 100g	0.2	374	40
Margarine, average	1 serving (10g)	0.1	75	8
	Per 100g	1	750	80
Margarine, Clover	1 serving (10g)	0	65	7
	Per 100g	0.2	654	72
Margarine, Flora	1 serving (10g)	0	78	8
	Per 100g	0.9	775	80
Margarine, soft	1 serving (10g)	0.1	73	8
	Per 100g	1	725	78
Margarine, Vitalite	1 serving (10g)	0.1	58	6
	Per 100g	1.2	578	63
Olive Oil spread, reduced fat	1 serving (10g)	0	50	6
	Per 100g	0.1	500	60
Unsalted low fat spread	1 serving (10g)	0	36	4
	Per 100g	0.9	360	35

FOOD	SERVING	CARBS (g)	CALS (kcal)	FAT (g)
Oils				
Blended oil	1 serving (25g)	0	196	24
	Per 100g	0	784	96
Coconut oil	1 serving (25g)	0	226	26
	Per 100g	0	905	105
Cod liver oil	1 serving (25g)	0	218	24
	Per 100g	0	870	95
Cottonseed oil	1 serving (25g)	0	220	25
	Per 100g	0	880	100
Corn oil, Mazola	1 serving (25g)	0	208	23
	Per 100g	0	830	92
Ghee, butter	1 serving (25g)	0	218	25
	Per 100g	0	870	100
Ghee, palm	1 serving (25g)	0	225	24
	Per 100g	0	900	95
Olive oil	1 serving (25g)	0	213	23
	Per 100g	0	850	90
Olive oil, extra virgin	1 serving (25g)	0	213	23
	Per 100g	0	850	92
Palm oil	1 serving (25g)	0	219	25
	Per 100g	0	875	100
Peanut oil	1 serving (25g)	0	219	26
	Per 100g	0	875	105
Rapeseed oil	1 serving (25g)	0	214	26
	Per 100g	0	855	105
Sesame oil	1 serving (25g)	0	216	26
	Per 100g	0	865	105
Sesame oil, organic	1 serving (25g)	0	225	26
	Per 100g	0	900	100
Soya oil	1 serving (25g)	0	234	25
	Per 100g	0	935	100
Sunflower oil	1 serving (25g)	0	225	26
	Per 100g	0	900	105

Calorie, Fat & Carbohydrate Counter

FOOD	SERVING	CARBS (g)	CALS (kcal)	FAT (g)
Vegetable oil	1 serving (25g)	0	226	25
	Per 100g	0	905	100
Wheatgerm oil	1 serving (25g)	0	235	25
	Per 100g	0	940	100

Condiments

Horseradish, prepared	1 tsp (16g)	1.3	5	tr
	Per 100g	8	31	0.1
Horseradish, raw	1 tsp (16g)	2.6	10	tr
	Per 100g	16	60	0.3
Olives, black	5 large (20g)	1.4	24	2.4
	Per 100g	7	120	12
Olives, green, unstuffed	5 large (18g)	0.3	27	2.9
	Per 100g	1.7	150	16
Pickles, dill	1 (about 60g)	2.7	12	0.1
	Per 100g	5	21	0.2
Pickles, sour	1 (about 30g)	0.8	4	0.1
	Per 100g	2.8	13	0.3
Pickles, sweet	1 (about 30g)	11	41	0.1
	Per 100g	35	140	0.3
Relish, sweet pickle	1 tsp (16g)	6	22	0
	Per 100g	37	140	0

Sauces

Apple chutney	1 tbsp (25g)	13	49	0.1
	Per 100g	50	195	0.2
Apricot chicken	1 serving (125g)	14	69	1
	Per 100g	11	55	0.8
Apricot chicken, jar	1 serving (125g)	18	69	10
	Per 100g	14	55	8
Baking powder	1 tbsp (25g)	9	43	0
	Per 100g	37	170	0
Barbeque	1 serving (30g)	10	41	0
	Per 100g	32	135	0

FOOD	SERVING	CARBS (g)	CALS (kcal)	FAT (g)
Barbeque sauce	1 tbsp (25g)	3.3	19	0.5
	Per 100g	13	75	1.8
Beef and black bean	1 serving (125g)	11	56	1.5
	Per 100g	9	45	1.2
Bolognaise	1 serving (125g)	3.4	188	14
	Per 100g	2.7	150	11
Bovril	1 tbsp (25g)	0.7	40	0.2
	Per 100g	2.8	160	0.7
Bread sauce, semi-skimmed milk	1 tbsp (25g)	3.3	23	0.8
	Per 100g	13	90	3
Bread sauce, whole milk	1 tbsp (25g)	3	28	1.3
	Per 100g	12	110	5
Brown sauce, bottled	1 tbsp (25g)	6	25	0
	Per 100g	24	100	0
Butterscotch	1 serving (45g)	14	218	16
	Per 100g	32	485	36
Cheese sauce packet mix, semi-skimmed milk	1 tbsp (25g)	2.5	23	0.9
	Per 100g	10	90	3.7
Cheese sauce packet mix, whole milk	1 tbsp (25g)	2.3	28	1.5
	Per 100g	9	110	6
Cheese sauce, semi-skimmed milk	1 tbsp (25g)	2.3	45	3.3
	Per 100g	9	180	13
Cheese sauce, whole milk	1 tbsp (25g)	2.3	48	3.8
	Per 100g	9	190	15
Chilli	1 serving (20g)	11	9	0
	Per 100g	55	45	0
Cook in sauce, canned	1 tbsp (25g)	2	11	0.2
	Per 100g	8	45	0.8
Country french chicken	1 serving (125g)	5	125	11
	Per 100g	4	100	9
Creamy lemon chicken	1 serving (125g)	15	69	0.8
	Per 100g	12	55	0.6
Creamy mushroom	1 serving (125g)	6	125	1.6
	Per 100g	5	100	1.3

Calorie, Fat & Carbohydrate Counter

FOOD	SERVING	CARBS (g)	CALS (kcal)	FAT (g)
Curry sauce, canned	1 tbsp (25g)	1.8	19	1.3
	Per 100g	7	75	5
French dressing	1 tbsp (25g)	0	163	19
	Per 100g	0.1	650	75
Gelatin	1 tbsp (25g)	0	84	0
	Per 100g	0	335	0
Golden honey mustard	1 serving (125g)	13	175	13
	Per 100g	10	140	10
Gravy instant granule, made with water	1 tbsp (25g)	0.8	9	0.6
	Per 100g	3	34	2.5
Gravy, commercial	1 serving (125g)	5	81	5
	Per 100g	4	65	4
Gravy, powder	1 serving (125g)	2.6	14	0
	Per 100g	2.1	11	0
Herbed chicken and wine	1 serving (125g)	8	14	6
	Per 100g	6	11	5
Honey and sesame	1 serving (125g)	23	113	1
	Per 100g	18	90	0.8
Honey, sesame and garlic	1 serving (125g)	23	81	0.5
	Per 100g	18	65	0.4
Horseradish sauce	1 tbsp (25g)	4	38	2
	Per 100g	17	150	8
Hungarian goulash	1 serving (125g)	8	106	3.4
	Per 100g	6	85	2.7
Malaysian satay	1 serving (30g)	5	69	5
	Per 100g	17	230	17
Mango chutney, oily	1 tbsp (25g)	13	70	2.8
	Per 100g	50	280	11
Marmite	1 tbsp (25g)	0.5	41	0.2
	Per 100g	1.8	165	0.7
Mayonnaise	1 tbsp (25g)	0.4	173	19
	Per 100g	1.7	690	75
Mild Indian	1 serving (125g)	8	88	8
	Per 100g	6	70	6

FOOD	SERVING	CARBS (g)	CALS (kcal)	FAT (g)
Mint sauce	1 tbsp (25g)	5	23	0
	Per 100g	21	90	0
Mint, homemade	1 serving (30g)	0	9	0
	Per 100g	0	30	0
Mornay, bought	1 serving (125g)	5	156	14
	Per 100g	4	125	11
Mustard, smooth	1 tbsp (25g)	2.5	34	2
	Per 100g	10	135	8
Mustard, wholegrain	1 tbsp (25g)	1	34	2.5
	Per 100g	4	135	10
Onion sauce, semi-skimmed milk	1 tbsp (25g)	2	23	1.3
	Per 100g	8	90	5
Onion sauce, whole milk	1 tbsp (25g)	2	24	1.8
	Per 100g	8	95	7
Onion, powder	1 serving (125g)	9	106	8
	Per 100g	7	85	6
Oxo cubes	1 tbsp (25g)	3	55	0.8
	Per 100g	12	220	3.3
Oyster	1 serving (30g)	5	30	0
	Per 100g	17	100	0
Packet sources, average	1 serving (125g)	10	263	21
	Per 100g	8	210	17
Pasta sauce, tomato based	1 tbsp (25g)	1.8	13	0.4
	Per 100g	7	50	1.5
Pesto	1 serving (30g)	9	90	5
	Per 100g	30	300	17
Pickle, sweet	1 tbsp (25g)	9	34	0.1
	Per 100g	34	135	0.3
Salad cream	1 tbsp (25g)	4	89	8
	Per 100g	16	355	31
Salad cream, reduced calorie	1 tbsp (25g)	2.3	50	4
	Per 100g	9	200	17
Salt, block	1 tbsp (25g)	0	0	0
	Per 100g	0	0	0

Calorie, Fat & Carbohydrate Counter

FOOD	SERVING	CARBS (g)	CALS (kcal)	FAT (g)
Salt, table	1 tbsp (25g)	0	0	0
	Per 100g	0	0	0
Soy sauce	1 tbsp (25g)	2	16	0
	Per 100g	8	65	0
Soya	1 serving (30g)	0.5	9	0
	Per 100g	1.7	31	0
Spicy plum	1 serving (125g)	21	88	0.5
	Per 100g	17	70	0.4
Sweet and sour	1 serving (125g)	29	125	0
	Per 100g	23	100	0
Sweet and sour, light	1 serving (125g)	19	81	0
	Per 100g	15	65	0
Sweet, Thai chilli	1 serving (125g)	56	194	0.5
	Per 100g	45	155	0.4
Toffee	1 serving (20g)	15	77	2
	Per 100g	75	385	10
Tomato	1 serving (30g)	5	23	0
	Per 100g	18	75	0
Tomato chutney	1 tbsp (25g)	10	43	0.1
	Per 100g	40	170	0.4
Tomato ketchup	1 tbsp (25g)	6	24	0
	Per 100g	20	95	0
Tomato sauce	1 tbsp (25g)	2.3	23	1.5
	Per 100g	9	90	6
Vinegar	1 tbsp (25g)	0.2	1	0
	Per 100g	0.5	3.9	0
White sauce semi-skimmed milk	1 tbsp (25g)	2.8	33	2
	Per 100g	11	130	8
White sauce, homemade	1 serving (30g)	2.4	26	5
	Per 100g	8	85	17
White sauce, sweet, semi-skimmed milk	1 tbsp (25g)	5	38	1.8
	Per 100g	20	150	7
White sauce, sweet, whole milk	1 tbsp (25g)	5	44	2.5
	Per 100g	19	175	10

FOOD	SERVING	CARBS (g)	CALS (kcal)	FAT (g)
White sauce, whole milk	1 tbsp (25g)	2.8	36	2.5
	Per 100g	11	145	10
Worcestershire	1 serving (30g)	4	17	0
	Per 100g	13	55	0
Yeast, bakers, compresses	1 tbsp (25g)	0.3	13	0.1
	Per 100g	1.1	50	0.4
Yeast, dried	1 tbsp (25g)	0.9	41	0.4
	Per 100g	3.7	165	1.4

Nuts

FOOD	SERVING	CARBS (g)	CALS (kcal)	FAT (g)
Almonds	1 serving (60g)	4	378	36
	Per 100g	7	630	60
Almonds, weighed with shells	1 serving (60g)	1.6	141	13
	Per 100g	2.6	235	21
Brazil nuts	1 serving (85g)	2.7	599	55
	Per 100g	3.2	705	65
Brazil nuts, weighed with shells	1 serving (85g)	1.3	281	26
	Per 100g	1.5	330	31
Cashew nuts, dry roasted, salted	1 serving (70g)	22	396	32
	Per 100g	32	565	45
Cashew nuts, dry roasted, unsalted	1 serving (70g)	23	417	32
	Per 100g	33	595	45
Cashew nuts, oil roasted, salted	1 serving (70g)	20	406	35
	Per 100g	28	580	50
Cashew nuts, oil roasted, unsalted	1 serving (70g)	21	413	35
	Per 100g	30	590	50
Chestnuts	1 serving (70g)	25	116	1.9
	Per 100g	36	165	2.7
Coconut, creamed block	1 serving (40g)	2.8	278	26
	Per 100g	7	695	65
Coconut, desiccated	1 serving (25g)	1.5	158	15
	Per 100g	6	630	60
Filberts, (hazelnuts) chopped	1 serving (70g)	10	434	46
	Per 100g	14	620	65

FOOD	SERVING	CARBS (g)	CALS (kcal)	FAT (g)
Hazelnuts	1 serving (70g)	4	434	46
	Per 100g	6	620	65
Hazelnuts, weighed with shell	1 serving (70g)	1.7	172	18
	Per 100g	2.4	245	25
Macadamia nuts, salted	1 serving (70g)	3.5	501	56
	Per 100g	5	715	80
Macadamia nuts, oil roasted, salted	1 serving (70g)	10	501	56
	Per 100g	14	715	80
Macadamia nuts, oil roasted, unsalted	1 serving (70g)	10	501	60
	Per 100g	14	715	85
Marzipan, homemade	1 serving (50g)	25	220	13
	Per 100g	50	440	26
Marzipan, retail	1 serving (50g)	35	195	7
	Per 100g	70	390	13
Mixed nuts	1 serving (70g)	6	441	35
	Per 100g	8	630	50
Mixed nuts w/ peanuts, dry, salted	1 serving (70g)	17	424	39
	Per 100g	24	605	55
Mixed nuts w/ peanuts, dry, unsalted	1 serving (70g)	18	413	39
	Per 100g	26	590	55
Mixed nuts w/ peanuts, oil, salted	1 serving (70g)	14	441	42
	Per 100g	20	630	60
Mixed nuts w/ peanuts, oil, unsalted	1 serving (70g)	15	455	42
	Per 100g	22	650	60
Peanut butter	1 tbsp (25g)	2.8	84	7
	Per 100g	11	335	28
Peanut butter, smooth	1 serving (50g)	7	310	28
	Per 100g	14	620	55
Peanuts, dry roasted	1 serving (70g)	7	406	35
	Per 100g	10	580	50
Peanuts, dry, roasted and salted	1 serving (70g)	5	410	35
	Per 100g	7	585	50
Peanuts, plain	1 serving (70g)	8	399	32
	Per 100g	12	570	45

FOOD	SERVING	CARBS (g)	CALS (kcal)	FAT (g)
Peanuts, plain, weighed with shells	1 serving (70g)	6	284	22
	Per 100g	9	405	31
Peanuts, oil roasted, salted	1 serving (70g)	13	431	35
	Per 100g	19	615	50
Peanuts, oil roasted, unsalted	1 serving (70g)	13	424	35
	Per 100g	18	605	50
Pecan nuts	1 serving (70g)	4	466	49
	Per 100g	6	665	70
Pine nuts	1 serving (25g)	1	178	18
	Per 100g	3.9	710	70
Pistachio nuts	1 serving (70g)	18	420	35
	Per 100g	25	600	50
Pumpkin and squash kernels	1 serving (70g)	13	396	32
	Per 100g	18	565	45
Sesame seeds	1 serving (40g)	0.4	250	24
	Per 100g	0.9	625	60
Sunflower seeds	1 serving (70g)	13	392	35
	Per 100g	18	560	50
Tahini	1 tbsp (25g)	2.8	83	7
	Per 100g	11	330	28
Tahini paste	1 serving (25g)	0.2	146	14
	Per 100g	0.9	585	55
Tofu	1 piece (10g)	1.1	32	1.8
	Per 100g	11	315	18
Walnuts	1 serving (70g)	2.3	462	49
	Per 100g	3.3	660	70
Walnuts, weighed with shells	1 serving (70g)	0.9	207	20
	Per 100g	1.3	295	28
Walnuts, black, chopped	1 serving (70g)	8	431	42
	Per 100g	11	615	60

Calorie, Fat & Carbohydrate Counter

FOOD	SERVING	CARBS (g)	CALS (kcal)	FAT (g)

MEAT

Beef

FOOD	SERVING	CARBS (g)	CALS (kcal)	FAT (g)
Beef liver, braised	1 serving (80g)	3	124	4
	Per 100g	3.6	155	5
Beef fat, cooked	1 serving (80g)	0	504	32
	Per 100g	0	630	65
Blade roast, lean only, braised	1 serving (160g)	0	384	21
	Per 100g	0	240	13
Bottom round roast	1 serving (160g)	0	336	13
	Per 100g	0	210	8
Brisket, lean only, braised	1 serving (160g)	0	384	21
	Per 100g	0	240	13
Brisket, boiled	1 serving (160g)	0	504	38
	Per 100g	0	315	24
Eye round roast, lean only	1 serving (160g)	0	272	8
	Per 100g	0	170	5
Filet mignon, lean only, broiled	1 serving (160g)	0	352	16
	Per 100g	0	220	10
Flank steak, lean only, broiled	1 serving (160g)	0	312	16
	Per 100g	0	195	10
Forerib, lean only, roast	1 serving (160g)	0	352	21
	Per 100g	0	220	13
Forerib, roast	1 serving (160g)	0	576	46
	Per 100g	0	360	29
Ground beef, extra-lean, broiled	1 serving (160g)	0	408	24
	Per 100g	0	255	15
Mince, stewed	1 serving (160g)	0	384	24
	Per 100g	0	240	15
Porterhouse steak, lean only, broiled	1 serving (160g)	0	344	18
	Per 100g	0	215	11
Pot roast, arm, lean only, braised	1 serving (160g)	0	352	13
	Per 100g	0	220	8

FOOD	SERVING	CARBS (g)	CALS (kcal)	FAT (g)
Rib eye steak, lean only, broiled	1 serving (160g)	0	360	19
	Per 100g	0	225	12
Rump steak, fried	1 serving (160g)	0	400	24
	Per 100g	0	250	15
Rump steak, grilled	1 serving (160g)	0	352	19
	Per 100g	0	220	12
Rump steak, lean only, fried	1 serving (160g)	0	312	11
	Per 100g	0	195	7
Shank cross cuts, lean only, simmered	1 serving (160g)	0	328	10
	Per 100g	0	205	6
Short ribs, lean only, braised	1 serving (160g)	0	480	29
	Per 100g	0	300	18
Silverside, lean and fat, salted	1 serving (160g)	0	368	22
	Per 100g	0	230	14
Silverside, lean only, salted and boiled	1 serving (160g)	0	280	8
	Per 100g	0	175	5
Sirloin steak, wedge bone, lean only, broiled	1 serving (160g)	0	320	11
	Per 100g	0	200	7
Sirloin, lean only, roast	1 serving (160g)	0	296	14.
	Per 100g	0	185	9
Sirloin, roast	1 serving (160g)	0	480	34
	Per 100g	0	300	21
Stewing steak, lean and fat, stewed	1 serving (160g)	0	368	18
	Per 100g	0	230	11
T-bone steak, lean only, broiled	1 serving (160g)	0	328	16
	Per 100g	0	205	10
Tip round steak, lean only, roasted	1 serving (160g)	0	288	11
	Per 100g	0	180	7
Top loin steak, lean only, broiled	1 serving (160g)	0	336	14
	Per 100g	0	210	9
Top round steak, lean only, broiled	1 serving (160g)	0	280	8
	Per 100g	0	175	5
Topside, lean and fat, roast	1 serving (160g)	0	336	19
	Per 100g	0	210	12

Calorie, Fat & Carbohydrate Counter

FOOD	SERVING	CARBS (g)	CALS (kcal)	FAT (g)
Topside, lean only, roast	1 serving (160g)	0	256	6
	Per 100g	0	160	3.9
Tripe, pickled	1 serving (160g)	0	96	2.1
	Per 100g	0	60	1.3

Lamb

FOOD	SERVING	CARBS (g)	CALS (kcal)	FAT (g)
Arm roast, lean only, roasted	1 serving (160g)	0	304	14
	Per 100g	0	190	9
Blade roast, lean only, roasted	1 serving (160g)	0	336	19
	Per 100g	0	210	12
Breast, lean and fat, roast	1 serving (160g)	0	656	58
	Per 100g	0	410	36
Breast, lean only, roast	1 serving (160g)	0	384	27
	Per 100g	0	240	17
Chops, grilled	1 serving (160g)	0	576	48
	Per 100g	0	360	30
Cutlets, grilled	1 serving (160g)	0	584	51
	Per 100g	0	365	32
Cutlets, grilled, weighed with bone	1 serving (160g)	0	376	30
	Per 100g	0	235	19
Cutlets, lean only, grilled	1 serving (160g)	0	344	19
	Per 100g	0	215	12
Foreshank, lean only, roasted	1 serving (160g)	0	304	10
	Per 100g	0	190	6
Ground lamb, broiled	1 serving (160g)	0	456	30
	Per 100g	0	285	19
Leg, lean and fat, roast	1 serving (160g)	0	424	29
	Per 100g	0	265	18
Leg, lean only, roast	1 serving (160g)	0	304	13
	Per 100g	0	190	8
Liver, braised	1 serving (80g)	2	184	7
	Per 100g	2.6	230	9
Loin roast, lean only, roasted	1 serving (160g)	0	304	16
	Per 100g	0	190	10

FOOD	SERVING	CARBS (g)	CALS (kcal)	FAT (g)
Loin, grilled, weighed with fat and bone	1 serving (160g)	0	200	11
	Per 100g	0	125	7
Rib roast, lean only, roasted	1 serving (160g)	0	360	21
	Per 100g	0	225	13
Scrag and neck, lean and fat, stewed	1 serving (160g)	0	488	32
	Per 100g	0	305	20
Scrag and neck, lean only, stewed	1 serving (160g)	0	400	26
	Per 100g	0	250	16
Shank, lean only, roasted	1 serving (160g)	0	272	11
	Per 100g	0	170	7
Shoulder, lean and fat, roast	1 serving (160g)	0	488	43
	Per 100g	0	305	27
Shoulder, lean only, roasted	1 serving (160g)	0	320	18
	Per 100g	0	200	11
Sirloin, lean only, roasted	1 serving (160g)	0	312	14
	Per 100g	0	195	9
Stew, lean only, broiled	1 serving (160g)	0	288	11
	Per 100g	0	180	7

Pork

FOOD	SERVING	CARBS (g)	CALS (kcal)	FAT (g)
Bacon rasher, fried, middle	1 serving (160g)	0	760	72
	Per 100g	0	475	45
Bacon rasher, lean, grilled	1 serving (160g)	0	456	29
	Per 100g	0	285	18
Bacon rasher, streaky	1 serving (160g)	0	688	64
	Per 100g	0	430	40
Bacon, Canadian	2 medium slices (about 45g)	0.6	86	3.9
	Per 100g	1.4	220	9
Bacon, collar joint, boiled	1 serving (160g)	0	496	45
	Per 100g	0	310	28
Bacon fat, cooked	1 serving (80g)	0	528	60
	Per 100g	0	660	75
Bacon, gammon joint, boiled	1 serving (160g)	0	392	30
	Per 100g	0	245	19

Calorie, Fat & Carbohydrate Counter

FOOD	SERVING	CARBS (g)	CALS (kcal)	FAT (g)
Bacon, gammon rasher, grilled	1 serving (160g)	0	368	19
	Per 100g	0	230	12
Bacon, gammon rasher, lean only, grilled	1 serving (160g)	0	264	8
	Per 100g	0	165	5
Bacon, ham, canned	1 serving (160g)	0	200	8
	Per 100g	0	125	5
Belly rashers, grilled	1 serving (160g)	0	664	58
	Per 100g	0	415	36
Blade loin roast, lean only, roasted	1 serving (160g)	0	464	29
	Per 100g	0	290	18
Center loin, lean only, roasted	1 serving (160g)	0	384	21
	Per 100g	0	240	13
Center rib, lean only, roasted	1 serving (160g)	0	376	22
	Per 100g	0	235	14
Chops, grilled	1 serving (160g)	0	520	40
	Per 100g	0	325	25
Chops, grilled, weighed with bone	1 serving (160g)	0	392	29
	Per 100g	0	245	18
Chops, loin only, grilled	1 serving (160g)	0	360	19
	Per 100g	0	225	12
Ham, cured, boneless roasted	1 serving (160g)	0.8	264	13
	Per 100g	0.5	165	8
Ham, fresh (leg), lean only, roasted	1 serving (160g)	0	352	18
	Per 100g	0	220	11
Leg, lean only, roast	1 serving (160g)	0	296	11
	Per 100g	0	185	7
Leg, roast	1 serving (160g)	0	440	34
	Per 100g	0	275	21
Liver, braised	1 serving (80g)	3	128	3
	Per 100g	3.7	160	4
Picnic shoulder arm, lean only, roasted	1 serving (160g)	0	376	21
	Per 100g	0	235	13
Pork fat, cooked	1 serving (80g)	0	508	32
	Per 100g	0	635	65

FOOD	SERVING	CARBS (g)	CALS (kcal)	FAT (g)
Shoulder blade, lean only, roasted	1 serving (160g)	0	392	26
	Per 100g	0	245	16
Sirloin, lean only, roasted	1 serving (160g)	0	392	21
	Per 100g	0	245	13
Spareribs, lean only, braised	1 serving (160g)	0	632	50
	Per 100g	0	395	31
Tenderloin, lean only, roasted	1 serving (160g)	0	264	8
	Per 100g	0	165	5
Top loin, lean only, roasted	1 serving (160g)	0	392	21
	Per 100g	0	245	13
Trotters and tails, salted, boiled	1 serving (160g)	0	472	34
	Per 100g	0	295	21

Poultry

FOOD	SERVING	CARBS (g)	CALS (kcal)	FAT (g)
Chicken drumsticks, broiler/fryer	1 serving (160g)	0	288	10
	Per 100g	0	180	6
Chicken leg, broiler/fryer	1 serving (160g)	0	328	14
	Per 100g	0	205	9.
Chicken wings, broiler/fryer	1 serving (160g)	0	320	13
	Per 100g	0	200	8
Chicken, boiled, meat only	1 serving (160g)	0	280	11
	Per 100g	0	175	7
Chicken, breaded, fried in oil	1 serving (160g)	26	341	19
	Per 100g	16	213	12
Chicken, leg quarter, roast, meat only	1 serving (160g)	0	152	6
	Per 100g	0	95	3.5
Chicken, meat and skin	1 serving (160g)	0	336	21
	Per 100g	0	210	13
Chicken, roast, meat only	1 serving (160g)	0	224	8
	Per 100g	0	140	5
Chicken, wing quarter, roast, meat only	1 serving (160g)	0	120	4
	Per 100g	0	75	2.6
Duck, roast, meat only	1 serving (160g)	0	312	16
	Per 100g	0	195	10

Calorie, Fat & Carbohydrate Counter

FOOD	SERVING	CARBS (g)	CALS (kcal)	FAT (g)
Duck, roast, meat, fat and skin	1 serving (160g)	0	560	46
	Per 100g	0	350	29
Goose, roast, meat, only	1 serving (160g)	0	520	35
	Per 100g	0	325	22
Grouse, roast, meat only	1 serving (160g)	0	264	8
	Per 100g	0	165	5
Grouse, roast, weighed with bone	1 serving (160g)	0	192	6
	Per 100g	0	120	3.6
Partridge, roast, meat only	1 serving (160g)	0	328	11
	Per 100g	0	205	7
Partridge, roast, weighed with bone	1 serving (160g)	0	208	6
	Per 100g	0	130	4
Pheasant, roast, meat only	1 serving (160g)	0	328	14
	Per 100g	0	205	9
Pheasant, roast, weighed with bone	1 serving (160g)	0	208	10
	Per 100g	0	130	6
Pigeon, roast weighed with bone	1 serving (160g)	0	168	10
	Per 100g	0	105	6
Pigeon, roast, meat only	1 serving (160g)	0	376	22
	Per 100g	0	235	14
Turkey, dark meat	1 serving (160g)	0	232	6
	Per 100g	0	145	3.9
Turkey, light meat	1 serving (160g)	0	216	2.2
	Per 100g	0	135	1.4
Turkey, meat and skin	1 serving (160g)	0	264	11
	Per 100g	0	165	7
Turkey, roast, meat only	1 serving (160g)	0	224	4
	Per 100g	0	140	2.8

Offal

FOOD	SERVING	CARBS (g)	CALS (kcal)	FAT (g)
Kidney, lamb, fried	1 serving (160g)	32	400	16
	Per 100g	20	250	10
Kidney, ox, stewed	1 serving (160g)	0	240	18
	Per 100g	0	150	11

FOOD	SERVING	CARBS (g)	CALS (kcal)	FAT (g)
Kidney, pig, stewed	1 serving (160g)	40	376	8
	Per 100g	25	235	5
Offal, tripe, dresses, stewed	1 serving (160g)	0	160	8
	Per 100g	0	100	5
Oxtail, stewed	1 serving (160g)	13	448	21
	Per 100g	8	280	13
Oxtail, stewed, weighed with bone	1 serving (160g)	8	192	14
	Per 100g	5	120	9
Heart, sheep, roasted	1 serving (160g)	0	448	29
	Per 100g	0	280	18
Heart, pig, stewed	1 serving (160g)	48	640	40
	Per 100g	30	400	25
Tongue, ox, boiled, fat removed	1 serving (80g)	0	260	21
	Per 100g	0	325	27
Tongue, sheep, stewed, fat removed	1 serving (80g)	0	240	20
	Per 100g	0	300	25
Tripe, dressed	1 serving (160g)	0	96	4
	Per 100g	0	60	2.6

Other meat

FOOD	SERVING	CARBS (g)	CALS (kcal)	FAT (g)
Hare, stewed, meat only	1 serving (160g)	0	312	13
	Per 100g	0	195	8
Hare, stewed, weighed with bone	1 serving (160g)	0	232	10
	Per 100g	0	145	6
Rabbit, stewed, meat only	1 serving (160g)	0	296	13
	Per 100g	0	185	8
Rabbit, weighed with bone	1 serving (160g)	0	144	6
	Per 100g	0	90	4
Veal, cutlet, fried in oil	1 serving (160g)	0	344	13
	Per 100g	0	215	8
Veal, fillet, roasted	1 serving (160g)	0	376	19
	Per 100g	0	235	12
Venison, roast	1 serving (160g)	0	304	10
	Per 100g	0	190	6

Calorie, Fat & Carbohydrate Counter

FOOD	SERVING	CARBS (g)	CALS (kcal)	FAT (g)

Cold meats *(values taken from Waitrose)*

FOOD	SERVING	CARBS (g)	CALS (kcal)	FAT (g)
Ardennes pate	Per pack (150g)	1.5	468	42
	Per 100g	1	312	28
Ardennes pepper salami	Per slice (7g)	0.1	30	2.7
	Per 100g	1.9	429	39
Bernard Matthew's chicken breast	Per slice (37g)	0.2	41	0.6
	Per 100g	0.6	110	1.5
Bernard Matthew's turkey breast	Per slice (37g)	0.2	42	0.6
	Per 100g	0.4	113	1.6
Bernard Matthew's premium Norfolk turkey breast	Per slice (20g)	0.5	20	0.2
	Per 100g	2.5	100	1.2
Black Forest ham	Per slice (7g)	tr	13	0.6
	Per 100g	0.6	181	8
Boiled ham	Per slice (13g)	tr	20	1
	Per 100g	tr	160	8
Bologna, beef	2 slices (about 60g)	0.4	76	16
	Per 100g	0.7	134	29
Bologna, Lebanon	2 slices (about 60g)	1.5	120	8
	Per 100g	2.6	212	13
Bologna, pork	2 slices (about 60g)	0.4	140	11
	Per 100g	0.7	247	20
Bologna, turkey	2 slices (about 60g)	0.6	113	9
	Per 100g	1.1	199	15
Bratwurst, fresh	1 link (about 85g)	1.8	256	22
	Per 100g	2.1	301	26
Breast of chicken	Per slice (13g)	0.2	20	1.1
	Per 100g	1.8	159	9
Brianca salami	Per slice (7g)	tr	24	1.8
	Per 100g	tr	348	26
Brussels pate	Per pack (150g)	1.5	489	45
	Per 100g	1	326	30
Chicken breast	Per slice (50g)	0.1	59	0.9
	Per 100g	0.1	119	1.8

FOOD	SERVING	CARBS (g)	CALS (kcal)	FAT (g)
Chicken liver pate	Per pack (113g)	3.3	370	35
	Per 100g	2.9	327	31
Chicken pate	Per pack (175g)	3.2	408	32
	Per 100g	1.8	233	18
Chicken roll, light meat	2 slices (about 60g)	1.4	90	4
	Per 100g	2.5	159	7
Chorizo, dried	1 link (about 60g)	1.1	273	23
	Per 100g	1.9	481	41
Corned beef	2 slices (about 60g)	0	142	9
	Per 100g	0	250	15
Country style pate with mushrooms	Per pack (150g)	1.5	489	45
	Per 100g	1	326	30
Crab pate	Per pack (113g)	0.6	236	19
	Per 100g	0.5	209	17
Duck pate	Per pack (175g)	16	488	39
	Per 100g	9	279	22
English ham	Per slice (12g)	tr	12	0.3
	Per 100g	0.3	97	2.5
English honey roast ham	Per slice (12g)	tr	18	0.8
	Per 100g	0.5	145	6
English smoked ham	Per slice (13g)	tr	18	0.8
	Per 100g	tr	140	6
Farmhouse selection oven baked chicken breast	Per pack (140g)	4	132	2.8
	Per 100g	1	94	2
Fiorucci – cubetti du pancetta	Per pack (140g)	0.9	448	36
	Per 100g	0.6	320	26
Fiorucci – pancetta arrodata	Per pack (80g)	0.3	212	16
	Per 100g	0.3	265	20
Frankfurter, beef	1 (about 45g)	0.8	142	13
	Per 100g	1.9	334	30
Frankfurter, chicken	1 (about 45g)	3.1	116	9
	Per 100g	7	273	21
Frankfurter, turkey	1 (about 45g)	0.7	102	8
	Per 100g	1.6	240	19

Calorie, Fat & Carbohydrate Counter

FOOD	SERVING	CARBS (g)	CALS (kcal)	FAT (g)
French country ham	Per slice (17g)	tr	22	0.8
	Per 100g	0.2	132	5
French garlic sausage	Per slice (13g)	0.1	27	2.1
	Per 100g	0.5	214	17
French ham and pistachio sausage	Per slice (12g)	0.1	33	2.9
	Per 100g	1	267	23
French salami	Per slice (5g)	0.1	22	1.8
	Per 100g	1.9	440	36
French saucisson sec with herbs de provence	Per slice (5g)	0.1	21	0.7
	Per 100g	1.9	421	13
Garlic pate	Per pack (150g)	1.5	468	42
	Per 100g	1	312	28
German Brunswick smoked sam	Per slice (20g)	0.1	32	1.8
	Per 100g	0.6	160	9
German extrawurst	Per slice (13g)	0.1	38	3.4
	Per 100g	0.8	303	27
German garlic rosette salami	Per slice (5g)	tr	17	1.3
	Per 100g	1.6	333	26
German pepper salami	Per slice (8g)	tr	26	2
	Per 100g	1	313	25
German roasted ham	Per slice (25g)	0..3	42	2.2
	Per 100g	1.1	169	9
German salami	Per slice (8g)	tr	28	2.2
	Per 100g	0.5	331	27
German strong garlic sausage	Per slice (5g)	tr	13	1.1
	Per 100g	0.8	253	21
Ham	2 slices (about 60g)	1.8	103	6
	Per 100g	3.2	182	11
Ham cubes	Per pack (100g)	0.2	145	5
	Per 100g	0.2	145	5
Hickory baked ham	Per slice (30g)	0.2	42	1.3
	Per 100g	0.7	140	4
Hickory smoked ham	Per slice (30g)	tr	44	1.4
	Per 100g	tr	146	5

FOOD	SERVING	CARBS (g)	CALS (kcal)	FAT (g)
Honey roast ham	Per slice (18g)	0.1	21	0.5
	Per 100g	0	118	3
Honey roast turkey breast	Per slice (20g)	0.2	21	0.2
	Per 100g	1.1	107	1
Italian dry cured ham	Per slice (13g)	tr	29	1.6
	Per 100g	0.2	221	12
Keilbasa, smoked	2 slices (about 60g)	1.2	176	15
	Per 100g	2.1	310	27
Knockwurst, smoked	1 link (about 70g)	1.2	209	19
	Per 100g	1.7	295	27
Liverwurst, fresh	3 slices (about 60g)	1.3	185	16
	Per 100g	2.3	326	29
Luxury Orkney crab pate	Per pack (100g)	9	178	11
	Per 100g	9	178	11
Milano salami	Per slice (5g)	tr	21	1.7
	Per 100g	tr	417	24
Mortadella	4 slices (about 60g)	1.8	187	15
	Per 100g	3.2	330	27
Oak smoked ham	Per slice (18g)	0.1	24	0.9
	Per 100g	0.4	135	5
Parma ham	Per slice (13g)	tr	37	2.5
	Per 100g	0.1	275	19
Pastrami slices	Per slice (10g)	tr	12	0.3
	Per 100g	tr	124	3
Pastrami, beef	2 slices (about 60g)	1.7	198	17
	Per 100g	3	349	29
Pastrami, turkey	2 slices (about 60g)	0.9	80	3.5
	Per 100g	1.6	141	6
Pepperoni	10 slices (about 60g)	1.6	273	24
	Per 100g	2.8	481	43
Pheasant pate	Per pack (175g)	5	382	30
	Per 100g	2.9	218	17
Porchetta	Per slice (25g)	tr	69	6
	Per 100g	tr	277	23

FOOD	SERVING	CARBS (g)	CALS (kcal)	FAT (g)
Prosciutto alle erbe	Per slice (31g)	tr	64	4
	Per 100g	tr	204	13
Riserva parma ham	Per slice (13g)	tr	33	1.9
	Per 100g	tr	247	15
Roast beef	Per slice (35g)	0.1	44	0.6
	Per 100g	0.3	125	1.8
Roast pork	Per slice (15g)	0.1	33	1.9
	Per 100g	0.3	221	12
Sage and onion turkey breast	Per slice (20g)	0.4	21	0.4
	Per 100g	2.2	105	2
Salami, beef	2 slices (about 60g)	1.6	148	12
	Per 100g	2.8	261	21
Salami, pork	3 slices (about 60g)	0.9	230	19
	Per 100g	1.6	406	34
Salami, turkey	2 slices (about 60g)	0.3	111	8
	Per 100g	0.5	196	14
Saucisson montague	Per slice (5g)	0.1	21	1.8
	Per 100g	1.9	421	37
Sausage, pork, fresh	4 links (about 60g)	0.5	192	16
	Per 100g	0.9	339	29
Scottish smoked wild venison	Per slice (20g)	0.4	41	2.1
	Per 100g	2	203	10
Serrano ham	Per slice (14g)	tr	28	1
	Per 100g	0.2	196	7
Smoked chicken breast	Per slice (20g)	0	28	1
	Per 100g	0	141	5
Smoked duck breast	Per slice (20g)	0.3	33	1.2
	Per 100g	1.6	165	6
Smoked mackerel pate	Per pack (113g)	1.1	390	36
	Per 100g	1	345	32
Smoked salmon pate	Per pack (113g)	1.7	245	18
	Per 100g	1.5	217	16
Smoked trout pate	Per pack (113g)	1.7	266	21
	Per 100g	1.5	235	18

FOOD	SERVING	CARBS (g)	CALS (kcal)	FAT (g)
Spanish chorizo	Per slice (5g)	0.1	15	1.2
	Per 100g	2	304	24
Spanish Serrano ham cubes	Per pack (150g)	0.3	294	11
	Per 100g	0.2	196	7
Tuna pate	Per pack (113g)	0.1	387	35
	Per 100g	0.1	342	31
Turkey breast	Per slice (55g)	0	65	0.9
	Per 100g	0	118	1.7
Turkey ham	2 slices (about 60g)	0.2	73	2.8
	Per 100g	0.4	129	5
Turkey roll, light meat	2 slices (about 60g)	0.3	83	4
	Per 100g	0.5	146	7
Venison pate	Per pack (175g)	8	583	51
	Per 100g	4	333	29
Wafer thin honey roast ham	Per slice (10g)	0.2	44	0.3
	Per 100g	1.5	440	2.6
Wafer thin honey roast turkey	Per slice (10g)	0.3	55	0.4
	Per 100g	3	550	4
Wafer thin honey smoked ham	Per slice (10g)	tr	41	0.2
	Per 100g	0.5	414	2.4
Wafer thin roast chicken	Per slice (10g)	0.3	55	0.5
	Per 100g	3	552	5
Wafer thin smoked turkey	Per slice (10g)	0.2	53	0.4
	Per 100g	1.6	527	4
Wild boar pate	Per pack (175g)	8	418	34
	Per 100g	4	239	19
Wiltshire cured honey roast gammon ham	Per slice (43g)	0.1	61	2
	Per 100g	0.2	142	5
Wiltshire mustard gammon ham	Per slice (43g)	0.1	62	2.2
	Per 100g	0.3	144	5
Wiltshire peppered gammon ham	Per slice (43g)	0.1	61	2.8
	Per 100g	0.3	142	6
Wiltshire smoked apple roast gammon ham	Per slice (43g)	0.1	62	1.9
	Per 100g	0.3	143	5

Calorie, Fat & Carbohydrate Counter

FOOD	SERVING	CARBS (g)	CALS (kcal)	FAT (g)
SOUP				
Asparagus (Covent Garden)	1 serving (250ml)	9	123	8
	Per 100ml	3.7	49	3.2
Autumn vegetable with mild spices (Baxter's Healthy Choice)	1 serving (250ml)	20	100	0.5
	Per 100ml	8	40	0.2
Beef and tomato (Batchelor's Original Cup-a-soup)	1 serving (250ml)	18	83	0.5
	Per 100ml	7	33	0.2
Beef consomme (Joubere Organic)	1 serving (250ml)	1.8	33	tr
	Per 100ml	0.7	13	tr
Bouillabaise (Spinnaker)	1 serving (250ml)	16	230	14
	Per 100ml	6	92	5
Broccoli and cauliflower (Batchelor's Slim-a-soup)	1 serving (250ml)	13	73	1.8
	Per 100ml	5	29	0.7
Cajun spicy vegetable (Batchelor's Slim-a-soup)	1 serving (250ml)	13	70	1.5
	Per 100ml	5	28	0.6
Cantonese hot and sour noodle soup (Campbell's Special Choice)	1 serving (250ml)	28	155	3.3
	Per 100ml	11	62	1.3
Carrot and butter bean (Baxter's)	1 serving (250ml)	20	138	4.8
	Per 100ml	8	55	1.9
Carrot and coriander (Baxter's)	1 serving (250ml)	14	95	3.5
	Per 100ml	6	38	1.4
Carrot and coriander (Knorr Vie)	1 serving (250ml)	10	95	5.5
	Per 100ml	3.9	38	2.2
Carrot and lentil (Heinz Weight Watchers)	1 serving (250ml)	15	78	0.3
	Per 100ml	6	31	0.1
Carrot, onion and chickpea (Baxter's Healthy Choice)	1 serving (250ml)	18	85	0.3
	Per 100ml	7	34	0.1
Cheese and broccoli with tagliatelle (Batchelor's Cup-a-soup Extra)	1 serving (250ml)	20	138	4.3
	Per 100ml	8	55	1.7

FOOD	SERVING	CARBS (g)	CALS (kcal)	FAT (g)
Chicken (Batchelor's Original Cup-a-soup)	1 serving (250ml)	15	115	6
	Per 100ml	6	46	2.2
Chicken (Campbell's Classics 99% Fat free)	1 serving (250ml)	13	85	2.3
	Per 100ml	5	34	0.9
Chicken (Heinz Weight Watchers)	1 serving (250ml)	10	75	2.5
	Per 100ml	4.1	30	1
Chicken and leek (Symington's soup in a cup)	1 serving (250ml)	15	123	6
	Per 100ml	6	49	2.5
Chicken and mushroom with pasta (Batchelor's Cup-a-soup Extra)	1 serving (250ml)	18	115	3.5
	Per 100ml	7	46	1.4
Chicken and sweetcorn (Batchelor's Slim-a-soup)	1 serving (250ml)	11	73	2.3
	Per 100ml	4.5	29	0.9
Chicken and vegetable (Batchelor's Cup-a-soup)	1 serving (250ml)	20	150	8
	Per 100ml	8	60	3
Chicken and white wine (Campbell's Classics – condensed)	1 serving (250ml)	10	123	8
	Per 100ml	4	49	3.3
Chicken broth (Baxter's Traditional)	1 serving (250ml)	13	90	1
	Per 100ml	5	36	0.4
Chicken noodle (Batchelor's Cup-a-soup)	1 serving (250ml)	18	105	2.3
	Per 100ml	7	42	0.9
Chicken noodle (Heinz Weight Watchers)	1 serving (250ml)	8	43	0.3
	Per 100ml	3.1	17	0.1
Chicken with vegetables (Baxter's Healthy Choice)	1 serving (250ml)	14	78	1.3
	Per 100ml	6	31	0.5
Chinese chicken noodle (Batchelor's Cup-a-soup Extra)	1 serving (250ml)	17	90	1
	Per 100ml	7	36	0.4
Chunky potato and leek with peppers and chicken (Stockmeyers Hearty Soups)	1 serving (250ml)	17	148	6
	Per 100ml	7	59	2.4

Calorie, Fat & Carbohydrate Counter

FOOD	SERVING	CARBS (g)	CALS (kcal)	FAT (g)
Chunky vegetable with pearl barley and lamb (Stockmeyers Hearty Soups)	1 serving (250ml)	12	113	2.8
	Per 100ml	4.7	45	1.1
Clam chowder (Spinnaker)	1 serving (250ml)	11	225	18
	Per 100ml	4.5	90	7
Cock-a-Leekie (Baxter's Traditional)	1 serving (250ml)	10	58	0.8
	Per 100ml	4.1	23	0.3
Country garden (Baxter's)	1 serving (250ml)	16	88	1.5
	Per 100ml	7	35	0.6
Country vegetable (Heinz Weight Watchers)	1 serving (250ml)	15	75	0.5
	Per 100ml	6	30	0.2
Country vegetable (Knorr Vie)	1 serving (250ml)	14	80	1.8
	Per 100ml	6	32	0.7
Courgette and crème fraiche (Baxter's fresh soup)	1 serving (250ml)	12	155	10
	Per 100ml	5	62	4.1
Cream of asparagus (Baxter's)	1 serving (250ml)	15	165	11
	Per 100ml	6	66	4.3
Cream of asparagus (Campbell's Special Choice)	1 serving (250ml)	12	113	7
	Per 100ml	5	45	2.8
Cream of chicken (Homepride)	1 serving (250ml)	10	113	7
	Per 100ml	4	45	2.9
Cream of chicken (Campbell's Classics – condensed)	1 serving (250ml)	9	120	9
	Per 100ml	3.5	48	3.6
Cream of mushroom (Campbell's Classics – condensed)	1 serving (250ml)	13	173	11
	Per 100ml	5.3	69	4.5
Cream of mushroom (Homepride)	1 serving (250ml)	9	110	8
	Per 100ml	3.5	44	3.1
Cream of tomato (Baxter's Traditional)	1 serving (250ml)	27	178	6
	Per 100ml	11	71	2.5
Cream of tomato (Campbell's Classics – condensed)	1 serving (250ml)	21	165	8
	Per 100ml	9	66	3.2

FOOD	SERVING	CARBS (g)	CALS (kcal)	FAT (g)
Cream of tomato (Homepride)	1 serving (250ml)	19	138	7
	Per 100ml	8	55	2.6
Creamy broccoli and cauliflower (Batchelor's Cup-a-soup)	1 serving (250ml)	16	108	4.3
	Per 100ml	6	43	1.7
Creamy potato and leek (Batchelor's Cup-a-soup)	1 serving (250ml)	19	118	3.8
	Per 100ml	7	47	1.5
Creamy potato bacon and onion (Batchelor's Cup-a-soup)	1 serving (250ml)	18	100	2.0
	Per 100ml	7	40	0.8
Creamy potato, leek and ham (Batchelor's Cup-a-soup)	1 serving (250ml)	17	98	2.3
	Per 100ml	7	39	0.9
Cullen skink (Baxter's)	1 serving (250ml)	15	190	13
	Per 100ml	6	76	5
French onion (Baxter's Traditional)	1 serving (250ml)	11	55	0.5
	Per 100ml	4.2	22	0.2
Gazpacho (Covent Garden)	1 serving (250ml)	11	88	3
	Per 100ml	4.2	35	1.2
Golden vegetable (Batchelor's Original Cup-a-soup)	1 serving (250ml)	18	83	0.5
	Per 100ml	7	33	0.2
Italian bean and pasta soup (Baxter's Healthy Choice)	1 serving (250ml)	18	95	0.5
	Per 100ml	7	38	0.2
Leek and potato (Joubere Organic)	1 serving (250ml)	15	123	6
	Per 100ml	6	49	2.4
Lentil and bacon (Baxter's Traditional)	1 serving (250ml)	20	150	4.8
	Per 100ml	8	60	1.9
Lentil and vegetable (Baxter's Healthy Choice)	1 serving (250ml)	17	90	0.3
	Per 100ml	7	36	0.1
Lobster bisque (Baxter's)	1 serving (250ml)	19	223	9
	Per 100ml	8	89	3.7

Calorie, Fat & Carbohydrate Counter

FOOD	SERVING	CARBS (g)	CALS (kcal)	FAT (g)
Mediterranean tomato and vegetable (Heinz Weight Watchers)	1 serving (250ml)	8	40	0.8
	Per 100ml	3	16	0.3
Mediterranean tomato (Batchelor's Slim-a-soup)	1 serving (250ml)	12	70	2
	Per 100ml	4.7	28	0.8
Mediterranean tomato (Baxter's fresh soup)	1 serving (250ml)	20	143	4.5
	Per 100ml	8	57	1.8
Minestrone (Batchelor's Cup-a-soup)	1 serving (250ml)	21	115	2.8
	Per 100ml	8	46	1.1
Minestrone (Baxter's Traditional)	1 serving (250ml)	15	85	1.5
	Per 100ml	6	34	0.6
Minestrone with croutons (Batchelor's Slim-a-soup)	1 serving (250ml)	11	65	1.5
	Per 100ml	5	26	0.6
Minestrone with pasta (Batchelor's Cup-a-soup Extra)	1 serving (250ml)	21	108	1
	Per 100ml	9	43	0.4
Minestrone with wholemeal pasta (Baxter's Healthy Choice)	1 serving (250ml)	17	80	0.5
	Per 100ml	7	32	0.2
Mushroom (Campbell's Classics 99% Fat free)	1 serving (250ml)	9	60	2.3
	Per 100ml	3.5	24	0.9
Mushroom potage (Baxter's)	1 serving (250ml)	13	103	16
	Per 100ml	5	41	6
Pea and ham (Baxter's Traditional)	1 serving (250ml)	20	145	4
	Per 100ml	8	58	1.6
Potato and leek (Baxter's Traditional)	1 serving (250ml)	20	110	2
	Per 100ml	8	44	0.9
Pumpkin (Covent Garden)	1 serving (250ml)	20	130	3
	Per 100ml	8	52	1.2
Red pepper and goats cheese (Covent Garden)	1 serving (250ml)	6	90	5
	Per 100ml	2.5	36	2.1

FOOD	SERVING	CARBS (g)	CALS (kcal)	FAT (g)
Rich woodland mushroom Batchelor's Cup-a-soup)	1 serving (250ml)	15	110	4.8
	Per 100ml	6	44	1.9
Scotch broth (Baxter's Traditional)	1 serving (250ml)	18	118	3
	Per 100ml	7	47	1.2
Scotch vegetable (Baxter's Traditional)	1 serving (250ml)	19	108	1.5
	Per 100ml	7	43	0.6
Seafood gumbo (Spinnaker)	1 serving (250ml)	13	208	12
	Per 100ml	5	83	4.8
Shropshire pea (Symington's soup in a cup)	1 serving (250ml)	18	103	2.5
	Per 100ml	7	41	1
Sicilian tomato (Covent Garden)	1 serving (250ml)	12	100	4
	Per 100ml	4.8	40	1.6
Spicy parsnip (Baxter's)	1 serving (250ml)	15	128	6
	Per 100ml	6	51	2.5
Spicy tomato and rice with sweetcorn (Baxter's Healthy Choice)	1 serving (250ml)	23	113	0.8
	Per 100ml	9	45	0.3
Spicy vegetable with noodles (Batchelor's Cup-a-soup Extra)	1 serving (250ml)	20	98	1
	Per 100ml	8	39	0.4
Spinach and nutmeg (Covent Garden)	1 serving (250ml)	11	73	1.5
	Per 100ml	4.5	29	0.6
Stilton and white port (Baxter's)	1 serving (250ml)	12	128	5
	Per 100ml	4.7	51	2.1
Sunrise soup (Covent Garden)	1 serving (250ml)	12	80	2.3
	Per 100ml	4.8	32	0.9
Tangy tomato with pasta (Batchelor's Cup-a-soup Extra)	1 serving (250ml)	23	120	2
	Per 100ml	9	48	0.8
Thai chicken and lemongrass (Batchelor's Cup-a-soup)	1 serving (250ml)	15	108	4.8
	Per 100ml	6	43	1.9

Calorie, Fat & Carbohydrate Counter

FOOD	SERVING	CARBS (g)	CALS (kcal)	FAT (g)
Thick and creamy tomato and basil (Batchelor's Cup-a-soup)	1 serving (250ml)	17	93	2.3
	Per 100ml	7	37	0.9
Tomato (Batchelor's Original Cup-a-soup)	1 serving (250ml)	20	100	1.8
	Per 100ml	8	40	0.7
Tomato (Heinz Weight Watchers)	1 serving (250ml)	12	63	1.3
	Per 100ml	4.6	25	0.5
Tomato and brown lentil (Baxter's Healthy Choice)	1 serving (250ml)	22	113	0.3
	Per 100ml	9	45	0.1
Tomato and orange (Baxter's)	1 serving (250ml)	21	108	1.3
	Per 100ml	8	43	0.5
Tomato and vegetable (Bachelor's Cup-a-soup)	1 serving (250ml)	19	130	4.5
	Per 100ml	8	52	1.8
Tomato, spinach and mascarpone (Covent Garden)	1 serving (250ml)	7	60	3
	Per 100ml	2.6	24	1.2
Vegetable (Campbell's Classics – condensed)	1 serving (250ml)	16	88	2
	Per 100ml	6	35	0.8
Wild mushroom	1 serving (250ml)	8	68	2.8
	Per 100ml	3	27	1.1

Tinned Soups

FOOD	SERVING	CARBS (g)	CALS (kcal)	FAT (g)
Cream of tomato (Heinz)	1 serving (250g)	18	160	9
	Per 100g	7	64	3.6
Beef and vegetables – Big Soup (Heinz)	1 serving (250g)	18	113	1.8
	Per 100g	7	45	0.7
Beef curry (Heinz)	1 serving (250g)	18	150	6.8
	Per 100g	7	60	2.7
Carrot and butterbean (Baxter's)	1 serving (250g)	20	138	4.8
	Per 100g	8	55	1.9
Chicken and vegetable (Heinz)	1 serving (250g)	16	95	2.3
	Per 100g	6	38	0.9
Chicken and vegetables – Big Soup (Heinz)	1 serving (250g)	18	118	2.5
	Per 100g	7	47	1

FOOD	SERVING	CARBS (g)	CALS (kcal)	FAT (g)
Chicken broth (Baxter's)	1 serving (250g)	13	75	1
	Per 100g	5	30	0.4
Country garden (Baxter's)	1 serving (250g)	16	88	1.5
	Per 100g	7	35	0.6
Cream of asparagus (Baxter's)	1 serving (250g)	15	165	11
	Per 100g	6	66	4.3
Cream of chicken (Campbell's)	1 serving (250g)	9	120	9
	Per 100g	3.5	48	3.6
Cream of chicken (Heinz)	1 serving (250g)	11	128	8
	Per 100g	4.4	51	3.2
Cream of mushroom (Campbell's)	1 serving (250g)	13	173	11
	Per 100g	5	69	4.5
Cream of mushroom (Heinz)	1 serving (250g)	13	128	7
	Per 100g	5	51	2.7
Cream of tomato (Campbell's)	1 serving (250g)	21	165	8
	Per 100g	9	66	3.2
Giant minestrone – Big Soup (Heinz)	1 serving (250g)	20	110	1.3
	Per 100g	8	44	0.5
Lentil (Campbell's)	1 serving (250g)	11	68	1.5
	Per 100g	4.3	27	0.6
Lentil (Heinz)	1 serving (250g)	19	103	0.5
	Per 100g	8	41	0.2
Lentil and vegetable (Baxter's)	1 serving (250g)	17	90	0.3
	Per 100g	7	36	0.1
Mediterranean tomato (Baxter's)	1 serving (250g)	17	83	0.5
	Per 100g	7	33	0.2
Minestrone (Baxter's)	1 serving (250g)	17	80	0.5
	Per 100g	7	32	0.2
Oxtail (Campbell's)	1 serving (250g)	13	105	3.8
	Per 100g	5	42	1.5
Oxtail (Heinz)	1 serving (250g)	17	100	1.5
	Per 100g	7	40	0.6
Potato and leek (Baxter's)	1 serving (250g)	20	110	2.3
	Per 100g	8	44	0.9

Calorie, Fat & Carbohydrate Counter

FOOD	SERVING	CARBS (g)	CALS (kcal)	FAT (g)
Potato and leek (Heinz)	1 serving (250g)	16	85	1.5
	Per 100g	7	34	0.6
Scotch broth (Baxter's)	1 serving (250g)	18	118	3.0
	Per 100g	7	47	1.2
Scotch broth (Heinz)	1 serving (250g)	20	118	1.8
	Per 100g	8	47	0.7
Tomato and orange (Baxter's)	1 serving (250g)	21	108	1.3
	Per 100g	8	43	0.5
Vegetable (Campbell's)	1 serving (250g)	16	88	2.0
	Per 100g	6	35	0.8
Vegetable soup (Heinz)	1 serving (250g)	21	118	2.3
	Per 100g	8	47	0.9

FOOD	SERVING	CARBS (g)	CALS (kcal)	FAT (g)

TINNED FOODS

Homepride cook in sauces

Chasseur sauce	390g tin	34	156	0.4
	Per 100g	9.2	40	0.1
Red wine sauce	390g tin	38	179	2.3
	Per 100g	9.8	46	0.6
Tomato and onion sauce	390g tin	39	187	2
	Per 100g	9.9	48	0.5
White wine and cream sauce	390g tin	33	301	18
	Per 100g	8.5	79	4.5

Tinned food

8 hot dogs (Tesco)	400g tin	20	732	58
	Per 100g	5	183	15
All day breakfast (HP)	415g tin	57	602	29
	Per 100g	14	145	7
Artichoke hearts (Tesco)	390g tin	23	121	0
	Per 100g	6	31	0
Baby carrots (Tesco)	300g tin	12	60	0.9
	Per 100g	3.9	20	0.3
Baby cobs (Green Giant)	220g tin	5	57	1.1
	Per 100g	2.4	26	0.5
Baked beans (HP)	420g tin	63	357	2.9
	Per 100g	15	85	0.7
Baked beans (Heinz)	415g tin	56	311	0.8
	Per 100g	14	75	0.2
Baked beans and pork sausage (Heinz)	415g tin	47	369	10
	Per 100g	11	89	2.5
Bamboo shoots (Amoy)	225g tin	22	88	0
	Per 100g	9.7	39	0
Beans in tomato sauce (Tesco)	420g tin	63	353	1.3
	Per 100g	15	84	0.3

Calorie, Fat & Carbohydrate Counter

FOOD	SERVING	CARBS (g)	CALS (kcal)	FAT (g)
Beef ravioli (Tesco)	200g tin	25	180	5.2
	Per 100g	12	90	2.9
Black eye beans (Tesco)	300g tin	59	354	2.4
	Per 100g	20	118	0.8
Borlotti beans (Tesco)	300g tin	48	309	2.1
	Per 100g	16	103	0.7
Broad beans (Tesco)	300g tin	34	255	2.1
	Per 100g	11	85	0.7
Butter beans (Tesco)	420g tin	46	302	2.1
	Per 100g	11	72	0.5
Cannellini beans (Tesco)	300g tin	53	330	3
	Per 100g	18	110	1
Celery hearts (Tesco)	400g tin	4.4	36	0.4
	Per 100g	1.1	9	0.1
Chestnut puree (Merchant Gourmet)	435g tin	118	579	8.7
	Per 100g	27	133	2
Chickpeas (Tesco)	400g tin	56	444	12
	Per 100g	14	111	2.9
Chicken and sweetcorn soup (Tesco)	200g tin	11	64	1
	Per 100g	5.3	32	0.5
Chicken hot curry (Tesco)	209g tin	14	257	13
	Per 100g	7	123	6.3
Chicken mild curry (Tesco)	209g tin	16	251	12
	Per 100g	8	120	5.6
Chilli beans (Tesco)	215g tin	47	249	1.5
	Per 100g	22	116	0.7
Chunky chicken in white sauce (Tesco)	206g tin	12	323	21
	Per 100g	6	157	10
Corned beef (Tesco)	340g tin	1.7	758	46
	Per 100g	0.5	223	14
Creamed mushrooms (Tesco)	200g tin	6.8	136	11
	Per 100g	3.4	68	5.5
Creamed style corn (Green Giant)	418g tin	50	238	2.1
	Per 100g	12	57	0.5

FOOD	SERVING	CARBS (g)	CALS (kcal)	FAT (g)
Curried beans (Heinz)	200g tin	36	406	2.6
	Per 100g	18	203	1.3
Extra crisp sweetcorn (Green Giant)	340g tin	45	238	2.4
	Per 100g	13	70	0.7
Fetch the vet spaghetti shapes (Heinz)	200g tin	18	148	7.1
	Per 100g	9	74	3.6
Garden peas (Tesco)	300g tin	28	201	2.7
	Per 100g	9.4	67	0.9
Giant marrowfat processed peas (Farrow's)	300g tin	37	231	1.5
	Per 100g	12	77	0.5
Glenrych's south atlantic pilchards (Glenrych's)	425g tin	9.8	485	18
	Per 100g	2.3	114	4.3
Green asparagus (Green Giant)	425g tin	8.5	68	0
	Per 100g	2	16	0
Healthy balance baked beans and vegetable sauce (Heinz)	400g tin	42	396	14
	Per 100g	10	99	3.6
Hot and spicy mixed beans (Tesco)	150g tin	20	117	0.8
	Per 100g	13	78	0.5
Italian chopped tomatoes (Tesco)	200g tin	8	46	0.4
	Per 100g	4	23	0.2
Italian chopped tomatoes and onion (Tesco)	200g tin	11	58	0.4
	Per 100g	5.7	29	0.2
Italian style mixed beans (Tesco)	300g tin	36	237	2.1
	Per 100g	12	79	0.7
Italiana – bolognaise shells (Heinz)	397g tin	38	282	5.2
	Per 100g	10	71	1.3
Italiana – tortellini (Heinz)	393g tin	33	232	7.2
	Per 100g	9	59	1.8
Jersey new potatoes (Tesco)	300g tin	41	186	0.3
	Per 100g	14	62	0.1
Kidney beans – no added salt or sugar (Tesco)	420g tin	63	391	2.5
	Per 100g	15	93	0.6

Calorie, Fat & Carbohydrate Counter

FOOD	SERVING	CARBS (g)	CALS (kcal)	FAT (g)
Leaf spinach (Tesco)	410g tin	14	116	1.2
	Per 100g	3.4	28	0.3
Lentil dahl (Tesco)	200g tin	21	248	13
	Per 100g	11	124	6.6
London grill (Heinz)	400g tin	43	404	12
	Per 100g	11	101	3.2
Lunch tongue (Tesco)	184g tin	0.6	318	19
	Per 100g	0.3	173	10
Macaroni cheese (Heinz)	201g tin	20	191	10
	Per 100g	10	95	4.7
Mackerel (Tesco)	125g tin	0	339	27
	Per 100g	0	271	21
Marrow fat processed peas (Batchelor's)	300g tin	41	234	0.9
	Per 100g	14	78	0.3
Marrowfat processed peas (Tesco)	300g tin	44	279	2.4
	Per 100g	15	93	0.8
Meat balls in bolognaise sauce (Campbell's)	410g tin	46	353	10
	Per 100g	11	86	2.5
Meat balls in gravy (Campbell's)	410g tin	35	328	11
	Per 100g	8.6	80	2.6
Meat balls in tomato sauce (Campbell's)	410g tin	39	340	11
	Per 100g	9.5	83	2.6
Mediterranean tomato, chicken and pasta soup (Tesco)	200g tin	15	80	1.1
	Per 100g	7.3	40	0.5
Mixed vegetables (Tesco)	300g tin	28	159	1.8
	Per 100g	9.2	53	0.6
Mushy peas (Tesco)	400g tin	45	300	2.8
	Per 100g	11	75	0.7
New potatoes (Tesco)	300g tin	42	186	0.3
	Per 100g	14	62	0.1
Pasta arrabbiata (Tesco)	206g tin	25	144	2.5
	Per 100g	12	70	1.2

FOOD	SERVING	CARBS (g)	CALS (kcal)	FAT (g)
Petit pois (Tesco)	397g tin	22	199	3.6
	Per 100g	5.5	50	0.9
Pink salmon (Tesco)	418g tin	0	552	31
	Per 100g	0	132	7.4
Pokemon (Heinz)	200g tin	22	176	6.2
	Per 100g	11	88	3.1
Prince's ham (Tesco)	454g tin	6.8	704	50
	Per 100g	1.5	155	11
Processed peas (Tesco)	300g tin	44	279	2.1
	Per 100g	15	93	0.7
Ratatouille provencale (Tesco)	390g tin	16	144	7
	Per 100g	4.2	37	1.8
Ravioli (Heinz)	200g tin	27	344	2.4
	Per 100g	13	172	1.2
Ravioli and tomato sauce (Tesco)	200g tin	28	138	0.2
	Per 100g	14	69	0.1
Red kidney beans (Tesco)	420g tin	63	391	2.5
	Per 100g	15	93	0.6
Red salmon (John West)	83g tin	tr	139	6.6
	Per 100g	tr	168	8
Red salmon (Tesco)	418g tin	0	660	42
	Per 100g	0	158	10.1
Rigatoni Carbonara (Tesco)	205g tin	22	236	11.9
	Per 100g	11	115	5.8
Sabrina spaghetti shapes (Heinz)	200g tin	24	120	0.8
	Per 100g	12	60	0.4
Sardines (Tesco)	120g tin	1.9	228	14.3
	Per 100g	1.6	190	12
Sild (John West)	110g tin	2.8	232	14.3
	Per 100g	2.5	211	13
Sliced button mushrooms (Tesco)	290g tin	1.7	32	0.58
	Per 100g	0.6	11	0.2
Sliced carrots (Tesco)	300g tin	13	66	0.9
	Per 100g	4.3	22	0.3

Calorie, Fat & Carbohydrate Counter

FOOD	SERVING	CARBS (g)	CALS (kcal)	FAT (g)
Sliced carrots – no added salt or sugar (Tesco)	300g tin	12	60	0.9
	Per 100g	3.9	20	0.3
Sliced green beans (Tesco)	300g tin	11	66	0.3
	Per 100g	3.8	22	0.1
Spaghetti (Heinz)	200g tin	26	122	0.4
	Per 100g	13	61	0.2
Spaghetti bolognaise (Heinz)	201g tin	25	159	3.2
	Per 100g	13	79	1.6
Spaghetti in tomato sauce (Tesco)	205g tin	26	123	0.4
	Per 100g	13	60	0.2
Spaghetti with chicken meatballs (Heinz)	200g tin	22	176	6.2
	Per 100g	11	88	3.1
Spaghetti with sausages (Heinz)	201g tin	22	165	5.2
	Per 100g	11	82	2.6
Spicy pasta spirals (Tesco)	200g tin	23	144	1.6
	Per 100g	12	72	0.8
Sweetcorn (Green Giant)	340g tin	71	340	1.1
	Per 100g	21	100	0.3
Sweetcorn (Tesco)	200g tin	31	164	2.2
	Per 100g	16	82	1.1
Tapper fillets (John West)	140g tin	tr	269	17
	Per 100g	tr	192	12
Teletubbies spaghetti shapes (Heinz)	203g tin	25	124	0.8
	Per 100g	12	61	0.4
Three bean salad (Tesco)	300g tin	53	330	3
	Per 100g	18	110	1
Tomato and orange soup (Tesco)	200g tin	14	66	0.4
	Per 100g	7	33	0.2
Tuna and onion (John West)	72g tin	2.9	101	3.6
	Per 100g	4	141	5
Tuna chunks (Tesco)	185g tin	0	350	17
	Per 100g	0	189	9
Tuna chunks (Tesco)	185g tin	0	361	19
	Per 100g	0	195	11

FOOD	SERVING	CARBS (g)	CALS (kcal)	FAT (g)
Unpeeled new potatoes (Tesco)	567g tin	79	363	1.7
	Per 100g	14	64	0.3
Vegetable broth soup (Tesco)	200g tin	15	74	0.4
	Per 100g	7	37	0.2
Vegetable ravioli (Tesco)	200g tin	33	164	1.4
	Per 100g	16	82	0.7
Water chestnuts (Amoy)	220g tin	22	92	0
	Per 100g	10	42	0
Whole button mushrooms (Tesco)	290g tin	1.7	32	0.6
	Per 100g	0.6	11	0.2
Whole green beans (Tesco)	400g tin	7	52	1.2
	Per 100g	1.6	13	0.3

2
Drinks

Calorie, Fat & Carbohydrate Counter

FOOD	SERVING	CARBS (g)	CALS (kcal)	FAT (g)
SOFT DRINKS				
Apple Juice	1 glass (240ml)	29	113	0
	Per 100ml	12	47	0
Apple juice, unsweetened	1 glass (240ml)	24	91	0
	Per 100ml	10	38	0
Apricot nectar	1 glass (240ml)	36	141	0.2
	Per 100ml	15	59	0.1
Bitter Lemon (Schweppes)	1 bottle (330ml)	28	115	0
	Per 100ml	8	35	0
Blackcurrant Juice, Ribena	1 carton (288ml)	40	164	0
	Per 100ml	14	57	0
Carrot juice	1 small glass (180ml)	17	74	0.3
	Per 100ml	9	41	0.2
Chocolate milk	1 glass (240ml)	26	208	9
	Per 100ml	11	87	3.8
Coca-Cola	1 can (330ml)	36	139	0
	Per 100ml	11	42	0
Cocoa, homemade	1 glass (240ml)	26	218	9
	Per 100ml	11	91	3.8
Cola, low-cal, with aspartame	1 can (330ml)	0.4	4	0
	Per 100ml	0.1	1.2	0
Cola, low-cal, with saccharin	1 can (330ml)	0.4	0	0
	Per 100ml	0.1	0	0
Cranberry juice cocktail	1 glass (240ml)	37	144	0.3
	Per 100ml	15	60	0.1
Cream soda	1 can (330ml)	45	172	0
	Per 100ml	14	52	0
Diet Coke	1 can (330ml)	0	1	0
	Per 100ml	0	0.3	0
Diet Fanta	1 can (330ml)	0.5	5	0
	Per 100ml	0.2	1.5	0
Diet Lemonade (Schweppes)	1 bottle (500ml)	0.2	8	0
	Per 100ml	0	1.6	0

FOOD	SERVING	CARBS (g)	CALS (kcal)	FAT (g)
Dry Ginger Ale (Schweppes)	1 can (330ml)	13	52	0
	Per 100ml	3.9	16	0
Eggnog	1 small glass (120ml)	17	171	10
	Per 100ml	14	143	8
Five Alive, Blackcurrant	1 carton (288ml)	44	180	0
	Per 100ml	15	63	0
Five Alive, Citrus	2 carton (288ml)	35	145	0
	Per 100ml	12	50	0
Five Alive, Orange Breakfast	3 carton (288ml)	31	133	0
	Per 100ml	11	46	0
Five Alive, Tropical	4 carton (288ml)	30	190	0
	Per 100ml	10	66	0
Five Alive, Very Berry	5 carton (288ml)	38	157	0
	Per 100ml	13	55	0
Fruit punch juice drink	1 glass (240ml)	30	124	0.5
	Per 100ml	13	52	0.2
Ginger Ale (Canada Dry)	1 can (330ml)	32	124	0
	Per 100ml	10	38	0
Grape juice drink	1 glass (240ml)	32	125	0
	Per 100ml	13	52	0
Grape juice, unsweetened	1 glass (240ml)	28	110	0
	Per 100ml	12	46	0
Grapefruit juice	1 glass (240ml)	22	79	0
	Per 100ml	9	33	0
Grapefruit juice, unsweetened	1 glass (240ml)	19	79	0
	Per 100ml	8	33	0
Lemon juice	1 glass (240ml)	3.8	17	0
	Per 100ml	1.6	7	0
Lemon-lime soda	1 can (330ml)	38	148	0
	Per 100ml	12	45	0
Lemonade from powder	1 glass (240ml)	25	97	0
	Per 100ml	10	40	0
Lemonade, bottled	1 glass (240ml)	14	50	0
	Per 100ml	6	21	0

Calorie, Fat & Carbohydrate Counter

FOOD	SERVING	CARBS (g)	CALS (kcal)	FAT (g)
Lemonade, white or pink	1 glass (240ml)	26	99	0.1
	Per 100ml	11	41	0
Lime juice cordial, undiluted	1 serving (50ml)	15	56	0
	Per 100ml	30	112	0
Limeade	1 glass (240ml)	27	101	0.1
	Per 100ml	11	42	0
Lucozade	1 glass (240ml)	43	161	0
	Per 100ml	18	67	0
Orange drink	1 glass (240ml)	32	126	0
	Per 100ml	13	53	0
Orange drink, undiluted	1 serving (50ml)	14	54	0
	Per 100ml	29	107	0
Orange juice	1 glass (240ml)	22	86	0
	Per 100ml	9	36	0
Orange soda	1 can (360ml)	46	179	0
	Per 100ml	13	50	0
Papaya nectar	1 glass (240ml)	36	143	0.4
	Per 100ml	15	60	0.2
Passion fruit juice	1 glass (240ml)	31	125	tr
	Per 100ml	13	52	tr
Peach nectar	1 glass (240ml)	35	135	tr
	Per 100ml	15	56	tr
Pineapple juice, unsweetened	1 glass (240ml)	26	98	0
	Per 100ml	11	41	0
Prune juice	1 glass (240ml)	45	182	0.1
	Per 100ml	19	76	0
Ribena, undiluted	1 serving (50ml)	30	114	0
	Per 100ml	61	228	0
Root beer	1 can (360ml)	39	152	0
	Per 100ml	11	42	0
Tea, iced, unsweetened, instant	1 glass (240ml)	0.5	2	0
	Per 100ml	0.2	0.8	0
Tomato juice	1 glass (240ml)	7	33	0
	Per 100ml	3	14	0

FOOD	SERVING	CARBS (g)	CALS (kcal)	FAT (g)
Tonic water	1 can (360ml)	32	124	0
	Per 100ml	9	34	0
Vegetable juice cocktail	1 glass (240ml)	10	46	0.2
	Per 100ml	4	19	0.1
Water, bottled	1 glass (240ml)	0	0	0
	Per 100ml	0	0	0
Water, municipal	1 glass (240ml)	0	0	0
	Per 100ml	0	0	0
Tea, brewed	1 cup (180ml)	0.5	2	0
	Per 100ml	0.3	1.1	0
Tea, herbal	1 cup (180m)	0.4	2	0
	Per 100ml	0.2	1.1	0

Calorie, Fat & Carbohydrate Counter

FOOD	SERVING	CARBS (g)	CALS (kcal)	FAT (g)
HOT DRINKS				
Banana flavour powder, made with semi-skimmed milk (Nestlé)	1 cup (200ml)	194	790	1
	Per 100ml	97	395	0.5
Bournvita powder, made with whole milk	1 cup (200ml)	15	152	8
	Per 100ml	8	76	3.8
Bournvita powder, made with semi-skimmed milk	1 cup (200ml)	16	116	3.2
	Per 100ml	8	58	1.6
Bovril chicken savoury drink	1 cup (200ml)	38	258	2.8
	Per 100ml	19	129	1.4
Cocoa powder (Cadbury's)	1 tbsp (15g)	1.7	52	3.3
	Per 100g	11	322	21
Cocoa powder, made with whole milk	1 cup (200ml)	14	152	8
	Per 100ml	7	76	4
Cocoa powder, made with semi-skimmed milk	1 cup (200ml)	14	114	3.8
	Per 100ml	7	57	1.9
Coffee, decaffeinated, black	1 cup (200ml)	0	0	0
	Per 100ml	0	0	0
Coffee Delight (Slim Fast)	1 cup (200ml)	22	132	1.6
	Per 100ml	11	66	0.8
Coffee, filtered, black	1 cup (200ml)	0.1	7	0
	Per 100ml	0.2	14	0
Coffee, ground, with 25ml ml full fat milk	1 cup (250ml)	2.5	23	1
	Per 100ml	5	46	2
Coffee, ground, with 25ml ml skim milk	1 cup (250ml)	2.5	18	0
	Per 100ml	5	36	0
Coffee, instant black	1 cup (200ml)	0	2	0
	Per 100ml	0	4	0
Coffee, instant, with 25ml full fat milk	1 cup (250ml)	1.5	18	1
	Per 100ml	3	36	2
Coffee, instant, with 25ml skim milk	1 cup (250ml)	1.5	13	0
	Per 100ml	3	26	0
Coffee, percolated, black	1 cup (200ml)	0.1	0	0
	Per 100ml	0.2	0	0

FOOD	SERVING	CARBS (g)	CALS (kcal)	FAT (g)
Coffee powder, percolator	1 cup (200ml)	0.6	4	0
	Per 100ml	0.3	2	0
Coffee powder, instant	1 tbsp (15g)	1.7	15	0
	Per 100g	11	100	0
Coffee and chicory essence	1 cup (200ml)	112	436	0.4
	Per 100ml	56	218	0.2
Coffeemate (Nestlé)	1 serving (7g)	4	36	2.1
	Per 100g	60	520	30
Drinking chocolate (Sainsbury's)	1 cup (200ml)	22	202	9
	Per 100ml	11	101	4.5
Drinking chocolate, made with whole milk	1 cup (200ml)	21	180	8
	Per 100ml	11	90	4
Drinking chocolate, made with semi-skimmed milk	1 cup (200ml)	22	142	3.8
	Per 100ml	11	71	1.9
Horlicks low fat instant powder	1 tsp (15g)	11	56	0.5
	Per 100g	73	373	3.3
Horlicks low fat instant powder, made with water	1 cup (200ml)	20	102	1
	Per 100ml	10	51	0.5
Horlicks powder, made with whole milk	1 cup (200ml)	25	198	8
	Per 100ml	13	99	3.9
Horlicks powder, made with semi-skimmed milk	1 cup (200ml)	26	162	3.8
	Per 100ml	13	81	1.9
Horlicks powder, made with skimmed milk	1 cup (200ml)	29	159	1.1
	Per 100ml	13	70	0.5
Irish coffee	1 cup (200ml)	0.1	189	10
	Per 100ml	0.2	378	20
Lift, Instant Lemon, reduced sweetness	Per pack (50g)	8.7	35	tr
	Per 100g	8.7	352	tr
Lift, Instant Lemon, original sweetness	Per pack (50g)	8.7	35	tr
	Per 100g	8.7	352	tr
Milk shake, purchased	1 cup (200ml)	26	180	6
	Per 100ml	13	90	3.2

Calorie, Fat & Carbohydrate Counter

FOOD	SERVING	CARBS (g)	CALS (kcal)	FAT (g)
Milk shake powder	1 tsp (15g)	15	58	0.2
	Per 100g	99	388	1.6
Milk shake powder, made with whole milk	1 cup (200ml)	22	174	7
	Per 100ml	11	87	3.7
Milk shake powder, made with semi-skimmed milk	1 cup (200ml)	23	138	3.2
	Per 100ml	11	69	1.6
Milky coffee (tsp coffee + 1 cup full fat milk)	1 cup (200ml)	12.5	173	10
	Per 100ml	25	346	20
Ovaltine powder	1 tsp (15g)	12	54	0.4
	Per 100ml	79	358	2.7
Ovaltine powder, made with whole milk	1 cup (200ml)	26	194	8
	Per 100ml	13	97	3.8
Ovaltine powder, made with semi-skimmed milk	1 cup (200ml)	26	158	3.4
	Per 100ml	13	79	1.7
Tea, Indian, infusion	1 cup (200ml)	0	0	0
	Per 100ml	0	0	0

London Fruit and Herb Company

Blackcurrant Bracer	Per pack (50g)	1	4	tr
	Per 100g	0.5	2	tr
Camomile and Honey	Per pack (50g)	0.4	2	tr
	Per 100g	0.2	1	tr
Fruit Burst Selection	Per pack (50g)	1	4	tr
	Per 100g	0.5	2	tr
Fruit Punch Selection	Per pack (50g)	1	4	tr
	Per 100g	0.5	2	tr
Pink Grapefruit Crush	Per pack (50g)	1	4	tr
	Per 100g	0.5	2	tr

FOOD	SERVING	CARBS (g)	CALS (kcal)	FAT (g)

ALCOHOL

Beers

FOOD	SERVING	CARBS (g)	CALS (kcal)	FAT (g)
Ale, brown, bottled	small (275ml)	8	82	0
	Per 100ml	3	30	0
Ale, pale, bottled	small (275ml)	6	77	0
	Per 100ml	2	28	0
Ale, strong	small (275ml)	17	182	0
	Per 100ml	6	66	0
Beer, average,	1 pint (574ml)	13	182	0
	Per 100ml	2.3	32	0
Beer, bitter, canned	1 can (440ml)	10	143	0
	Per 100ml	2.3	33	0
Beer, bitter, canned	large (500ml)	12	161	0
	Per 100ml	2.3	32	0
Beer, bitter, low alcohol	1 pint (574ml)	12	75	0
	Per 100ml	2.1	13	0
Beer, draught	1 pint (574ml)	13	184	0
	Per 100ml	2.3	32	0
Beer, keg	1 pint (574ml)	13	178	0
	Per 100ml	2.3	31	0
Beer, mild, draught	small (275ml)	9	145	0
	Per 100ml	3.4	53	0
Lager, bottled	large (500ml)	8	146	0
	Per 100ml	1.5	29	0
Lager, reduced alcohol	1 pint (574ml)	9	57	0
	Per 100ml	1.5	10	0
Shandy, canned	large (500ml)	15	55	0
	Per 100ml	3	11	0
Stout, bottled	small (275ml)	11	100	0
	Per 100ml	4	36	0
Stout, strong	large (500ml)	11	195	0
	Per 100ml	2.1	39	0

Calorie, Fat & Carbohydrate Counter

FOOD	SERVING	CARBS (g)	CALS (kcal)	FAT (g)
Stout, strong	small (275ml)	6	107	0
	Per 100ml	2.1	39	0

Ciders

FOOD	SERVING	CARBS (g)	CALS (kcal)	FAT (g)
Cider, dry	1 pint (574ml)	15	208	0
	Per 100ml	2.6	36	0
Cider, sweet	1 pint (574ml)	24	244	0
	Per 100ml	4	43	0
Cider, vintage, strong	1 pint (574ml)	42	578	0
	Per 100ml	7	101	0

Cocktails

FOOD	SERVING	CARBS (g)	CALS (kcal)	FAT (g)
Cocktail, Bloody Mary	1 glass (240ml)	8	180	0
	Per 100ml	3.3	75	0
Cocktail, Daiquiri	1 glass (240ml)	17	444	0
	Per 100ml	7	185	0
Cocktail, Daiquiri – canned	1 can (204ml)	32	259	0
	Per 100ml	16	127	0
Cocktail, Tequila Sunrise	1 glass (240ml)	29	158	0
	Per 100ml	12	110	0
Cocktail, Tequila sunrise – can	1 can (204ml)	24	232	0
	Per 100ml	12	114	0

Liqueurs

FOOD	SERVING	CARBS (g)	CALS (kcal)	FAT (g)
Coffee liqueur 53 proof	1 shot (30ml)	16	117	0
	Per 100ml	53	390	0
Coffee liqueur 63 proof	1 shot (30ml)	11	107	0
	Per 100ml	37	357	0
Coffee liqueur + cream	1 shot (30ml)	6	102	5
	Per 100ml	20	340	17
Liqueur, egg-based	1 shot (25ml)	7	65	0
	Per 100ml	28	260	0
Liqueur, cherry brandy/coffee	1 shot (25ml)	8	66	0
	Per 100ml	33	262	0

FOOD	SERVING	CARBS (g)	CALS (kcal)	FAT (g)
Liqueur, cream	1 shot (25ml)	6	81	0
	Per 100ml	24	324	0
Liqueur, drambuie	1 shot (25ml)	6	79	0
	Per 100ml	24	314	0

Spirits

Brandy, average, 40% volume	1 shot (25ml)	0	55	0
	Per 100ml	0	220	0
Gin and tonic	1 glass (240ml)	17	182	0
	Per 100ml	7	76	0
Gin,	1 shot (30ml)	0	73	0
	Per 100ml	0	243	0
Gin, average, 40% volume	1 shot (25ml)	0	55	0
	Per 100ml	0	220	0
Manhattan	30ml	2	128	0
	Per 100ml	3.3	213	0
Martini	30ml	0	156	0
	Per 100ml	0	208	0
Rum	1 shot (30ml)	0	64	0
	Per 100ml	0	213	0
Rum, average, 40% volume	1 shot (25ml)	0	55	0
	Per 100ml	0	220	0
Screwdriver	1 glass (240ml)	22	199	0
	Per 100ml	9	83	0
Spirits, average, 37.5% volume	1 shot (25ml)	0	51	0
	Per 100ml	0	204	0
Vodka, average, 40% volume	1 shot (25ml)	0	55	0
	Per 100ml	0	220	0
Whisky, average, 40% volume	1 shot (25ml)	0	55	0
	Per 100ml	0	220	0

Wine

Champagne	1 small glass (125ml)	1.7	95	0
	Per 100ml	1.4	76	0

Calorie, Fat & Carbohydrate Counter

FOOD	SERVING	CARBS (g)	CALS (kcal)	FAT (g)
Dessert wine – dry	1 shot glass (30ml)	1	38	0
	Per 100ml	3.3	127	0
Dessert wine – sweet	1 shot glass 30ml)	4	46	0
	Per 100ml	13	153	0
Red wine	1 glass (125ml)	2.4	168	0
	Per 100ml	1.9	70	0
Wine, fortified, port	1 shot glass (50ml)	6	80	0
	Per 100ml	12	160	0
Wine, fortified, sherry, dry	1 shot glass (50ml)	0.7	58	0
	Per 100ml	1.4	116	0
Wine, fortified, sherry, medium	1 shot glass (50ml)	3	60	0
	Per 100ml	6	120	0
Wine , fortified, sherry, sweet	1 shot glass (50ml)	3.5	68	0
	Per 100ml	7	136	0
Wine , fortified, vermouth, dry	1 shot glass (50ml)	1.5	55	0
	Per 100ml	3	110	0
Wine , fortified, vermouth, sweet	1 shot glass (50ml)	8	75	0
	Per 100ml	15	150	0
Wine, red	1 small glass (120ml)	0.4	85	0
	Per 100ml	0.3	71	0
Wine , rose	1 small glass (120ml)	3.1	89	0
	Per 100ml	2.6	74	0
Wine , white, dry	1 small glass (120ml)	0.7	82	0
	Per 100ml	0.6	68	0
Wine , white, medium	1 small glass (120ml)	4	94	0
	Per 100ml	3.6	78	0
Wine , white, sweet	1 small glass (120ml)	7	118	0
	Per 100ml	6	98	0

3
Breakfast foods

Calorie, Fat & Carbohydrate Counter

FOOD	SERVING	CARBS (g)	CALS (kcal)	FAT (g)
Cereals				
All-Bran (Kellogg's)	Per bowl (about 30g)	14	81	1.2
	Per 100g	46	270	4
Alpen (Weetabix)	Per bowl (30g)	20	110	2.1
	Per 100g	66	365	7
Bran Flakes (Kellogg's)	Per bowl (30g)	20	96	0.9
	Per 100g	66	320	3
Cheerios (Nestlé)	Per bowl (30g)	23	111	1.2
	Per 100g	75	369	4
Cinnamon Grahams (Nestlé)	Per bowl (30g)	23	125	3.3
	Per 100g	76	416	11
Coco Pops (Kellogg's)	Per bowl (30g)	26	114	0.9
	Per 100g	85	380	3
Corn Flakes (Kellogg's)	Per bowl (30g)	25	111	0.3
	Per 100g	83	370	1
Country Store (Kellogg's)	Per bowl (30g)	21	108	1.5
	Per 100g	69	360	5
Crunchy Nut Cornflakes (Kellogg's)	Per bowl (30g)	25	117	1.2
	Per 100g	83	390	4
Frosted Shreddies (Nestlé)	Per bowl (30g)	24	107	0.3
	Per 100g	81	356	1
Frosties (Kellogg's)	Per bowl (30g)	26	111	0.3
	Per 100g	87	370	1
Fruit 'n' Fibre (Kellogg's)	Per bowl (30g)	21	105	1.5
	Per 100g	71	350	5
Golden Grahams (Nestlé)	Per bowl (30g)	24	114	1.2
	Per 100g	81	381	4
Golden Nuggets (Nestlé)	Per bowl (30g)	26	118	0.9
	Per 100g	87	392	3
Harvest Crunch (Quaker)	Per bowl (30g)	19	131	5
	Per 100g	63	437	17
Honey Nut Cheerios (Nestlé)	Per bowl (30g)	23	112	0.9
	Per 100g	78	374	3

FOOD	SERVING	CARBS (g)	CALS (kcal)	FAT (g)
Multi-Grain Start (Kellogg's)	Per bowl (30g)	24	108	0.6
	Per 100g	81	360	2
Natural Muesli (Jordan's)	Per bowl (30g)	19	106	2.1
	Per 100g	62	352	7
Nesquick (Nestlé)	Per bowl (30g)	26	119	1.5
	Per 100g	85	398	5
Porridge, made with milk	Per bowl (30g)	4	35	1.5
	Per 100g	14	115	5
Porridge, made with water	Per bowl (30g)	2.7	15	0.3
	Per 100g	9	50	1
Quaker Puffed Wheat (Quaker)	Per bowl (30g)	19	98	0.3
	Per 100g	62	328	1
Ready Brek (Weetabix)	Per bowl (30g)	7	107	2.4
	Per 100g	24	356	8
Ready Brek Chocolate (Weetabix)	Per bowl (30g)	18	108	2.1
	Per 100g	60	360	7
Rice Krispies (Kellogg's)	Per bowl (30g)	26	111	0.3
	Per 100g	87	370	1
Ricicles (Kellogg's)	Per bowl (30g)	27	114	0.3
	Per 100g	89	380	1
Shredded Wheat	Per bowl (30g)	20	99	0.6
	Per 100g	66	330	2
Shreddies	Per bowl (30g)	22	103	0.6
	Per 100g	72	343	2
Special K (Kellogg's)	Per bowl (30g)	23	111	0.3
	Per 100g	76	370	1
Sugar Puffs (Quaker)	Per bowl (30g)	26	116	0.3
	Per 100g	85	387	1
Sultana Bran (Kellogg's)	Per bowl (30g)	20	96	0.6
	Per 100g	66	320	2
Weetabix (Weetabix)	Per bowl (30g)	20	102	0.9
	Per 100g	68	340	3
Weetos (Weetabix)	Per bowl (30g)	23	115	1.5
	Per 100g	78	384	5

Calorie, Fat & Carbohydrate Counter

FOOD	SERVING	CARBS (g)	CALS (kcal)	FAT (g)
Breakfast foods				
Biscuit w/ egg and bacon	1 (about 150g)	29	462	32
	Per 100g	19	308	21
Biscuit w/ egg and ham	1 (about 200g)	30	446	28
	Per 100g	15	223	14
Biscuit w/ egg and sausage	1 (about 200g)	42	586	40
	Per 100g	21	293	20
Biscuit with egg, cheese, and bacon	1 (about 140g)	34	472	31
	Per 100g	24	337	22
Croissant with egg and cheese	1 (about 130g)	25	374	25
	Per 100g	19	288	19
Croissant with egg, cheese, and bacon	1 (about 130g)	25	421	36
	Per 100g	19	324	28
Croissant with egg, cheese, and ham	1 (about 155g)	25	471	34
	Per 100g	16	304	22
Croissant with egg, cheese, and sausage	1 (about 165g)	25	530	38
	Per 100g	15	321	23
Danish pastry, cheese	1 (about 90g)	28	345	24
	Per 100g	31	383	27
Danish pastry, cinnamon	1 (about 85g)	47	349	17
	Per 100g	55	410	20
Danish pastry, fruit	1 (about 90g)	44	328	15
	Per 100g	49	364	17
English muffin w/egg, cheese, & sausage	1 (about 170g)	31	486	31
	Per 100g	18	286	18
French toast sticks	5 (about 140g)	49	472	29
	Per 100g	35	337	21

4
Lunchtime foods

Calorie, Fat & Carbohydrate Counter

FOOD	SERVING	CARBS (g)	CALS (kcal)	FAT (g)
Snack foods				
Burger rings	1 packet (50g)	0	249	13
	Per 100g	0	498	26
Cheese twists	1 packet (50g)	30	249	13
	Per 100g	60	498	26
Cheese potato puffs	1 packet (50g)	30	258	15
	Per 100g	60	516	30
Popcorn, microwave	1 packet (50g)	25	249	15
	Per 100g	50	498	30
Potato crisps	1 packet (50g)	30	258	15
	Per 100g	60	516	30
Pork rind, crackling	1 packet (30g)	0	45	2
	Per 100g	0	150	7
Prawn crackers	1 packet (10g)	7	37	0.5
	Per 100g	65	370	5
Pretzel	1 packet (45g)	20	167	12
	Per 100g	44	371	27
Crisps				
Doritos, cool original	1 packet (35g)	22	179	9
	Per 100g	62	510	26
Doritos, Dippa, hint of garlic	1 packet (35g)	21	173	9
	Per 100g	60	495	25
Doritos, Dippa, lightly salted	1 packet (35g)	22	172	8
	Per 100g	63	490	23
Doritos, Dippa, lime	1 packet (35g)	21	173	9
	Per 100g	60	495	25
Frisps, cheese and onion	1 packet (28g)	15	150	9
	Per 100g	53	537	34
Frisps, ready salted	1 packet (28g)	15	151	10
	Per 100g	52	541	35
Frisps, salt and vinegar	1 packet (28g)	14	144	9
	Per 100g	51	513	32

FOOD	SERVING	CARBS (g)	CALS (kcal)	FAT (g)
Golden Wonder, Wheat Crunchies, BBQ	1 packet (25g)	15	135	8
	Per 100g	60	539	32
Golden Wonder, Wheat Crunchies, cheese	1 packet (25g)	14	138	8
	Per 100g	57	550	34
Golden Wonder, Wheat Crunchies, crispy bacon	1 packet (35g)	20	172	9
	Per 100g	56	491	25
Hula hoops, original	1 packet (27g)	15	140	8
	Per 100g	55	517	31
Jacobs, Twiglets, original	1 packet (125g)	77	488	14
	Per 100g	61	390	11
Kettle chips, lightly salted	1 packet (50g)	26	233	13
	Per 100g	52	465	26
Kettle chips, New York cheddar	1 packet (50g)	27	242	13
	Per 100g	54	483	27
Kettle chips, salsa and mesquite	1 packet (50g)	12	229	12
	Per 100g	24	458	24
Kettle chips, sea salt and balsamic vinegar	1 packet (50g)	30	234	12
	Per 100g	61	468	24
Kettle chips, sea salt and crushed black pepper	1 packet (50g)	27	239	13
	Per 100g	53	477	26
McCoys, flame steak grilled	1 packet (50g)	27	252	15
	Per 100g	54	504	29
McVitie's, Mini Cheddars	1 packet (50g)	27	268	15
	Per 100g	54	535	30
Pringles, cheese and onion	1 packet (200g)	98	1088	72
	Per 100g	49	544	36
Pringles, curry	1 packet (200g)	92	1062	72
	Per 100g	46	531	36
Pringles, hot and spicy	1 packet (200g)	98	1092	74
	Per 100g	49	546	37
Pringles, original	1 packet (200g)	96	1114	76
	Per 100g	48	557	38
Pringles, salt and vinegar	1 packet (200g)	100	1090	72
	Per 100g	50	545	36

Calorie, Fat & Carbohydrate Counter

FOOD	SERVING	CARBS (g)	CALS (kcal)	FAT (g)
Pringles, sour cream and onion	1 packet (200g)	98	1100	74
	Per 100g	48	550	37
Pringles, Texas, BBQ sauce	1 packet (200g)	100	1088	76
	Per 100g	50	544	36
Symington's, chicken and leek	1 packet (224g)	13	110	6
	Per 100g	6	49	2.5
Symington's, shropshire pea	1 packet (100g)	7.2	95	2.2
	Per 100g	7.2	95	2.2
Walkers Max, chargrilled steak	1 packet (55g)	28	289	18
	Per 100g	50	525	33
Walkers Max, cheese and onion	1 packet (55g)	28	289	18
	Per 100g	50	525	33
Walkers Max, chip shop curry	1 packet (55g)	28	289	18
	Per 100g	50	525	33
Walkers Quavers,	1 packet (20g)	12	103	6
	Per 100g	61	515	29
Walkers, barbeque	1 packet (25g)	13	131	8
	Per 100g	50	525	33
Walkers, cheese and onion	1 packet (34g)	17	179	11
	Per 100g	50	525	33
Walkers, French Fries, salt and vinegar	1 packet (22g)	14	92	3.5
	Per 100g	63	420	16
Walkers, Monster Munch, cheese and onion	1 packet (28g)	17	130	6
	Per 100g	61	465	21
Walkers, Monster Munch, pickled onion	1 packet (25g)	14	120	6
	Per 100g	57	480	25
Walkers, Monster Munch, ready salted	1 packet (28g)	6	132	6
	Per 100g	22	470	22
Walkers, Monster Munch, salt and vinegar	1 packet (28g)	17	130	6
	Per 100g	61	465	21
Walkers, prawn cocktail	1 packet (34g)	17	179	11
	Per 100g	50	525	33
Walkers, prawn skips	1 packet (34g)	20	176	10
	Per 100g	60	517	29

FOOD	SERVING	CARBS (g)	CALS (kcal)	FAT (g)
Walkers, ready salted	1 packet (34g)	17	186	12
	Per 100g	49	530	34
Walkers, roast chicken	1 packet (34g)	17	179	11
	Per 100g	50	525	33
Walkers, salt and vinegar	1 packet (34g)	17	179	11
	Per 100g	50	525	33
Walkers, smokey bacon	1 packet (34g)	17	179	11
	Per 100g	50	525	33
Walkers, tomato ketchup	1 packet (34g)	18	180	11
	Per 100g	50	515	32
Wotsits, cheesy flavour	1 packet (21g)	11	114	7
	Per 100g	51	541	34

Salads

FOOD	SERVING	CARBS (g)	CALS (kcal)	FAT (g)
Greek	30g	0.5	39	3.8
	Per 100g	1.9	130	13
Green	30g	0.5	3.2	0.1
	Per 100g	1.8	12	0.3
Pasta	30g	4	39	2.3
	Per 100g	13	127	7
Pasta, wholemeal	30g	4.2	40	2.3
	Per 100g	14	131	8
Potato with french dressing	30g	4.1	47	3.3
	Per 100g	14	157	11
Potato with mayonnaise	30g	3.6	72	6
	Per 100g	12	239	21
Rice	30g	7	49	2.3
	Per 100g	23	166	8
Rice, brown	30g	7	50	2.3
	Per 100g	24	167	7
Tomato & onion	30g	1.2	21	1.8
	Per 100g	4	72	6
Waldorf	30g	2.3	58	5
	Per 100g	8	193	18

Calorie, Fat & Carbohydrate Counter

FOOD	SERVING	CARBS (g)	CALS (kcal)	FAT (g)

Tesco – salads

FOOD	SERVING	CARBS (g)	CALS (kcal)	FAT (g)
Alfresco style	1 pack (250g)	8	50	0.8
	Per 100g	3.3	20	0.3
Baby leaf with watercress	1 pack (110g)	1.4	21	0.8
	Per 100g	1.3	19	0.7
Baby leaf with watercress	1 pack (110g)	1.4	21	0.8
	Per 100g	1.3	19	0.7
Basil and parmesan pasta salad	1 pack (200g)	40	260	7
	Per 100g	20	130	3.6
Caesar salad	1 pack (295g)	20	466	39
	Per 100g	7	158	13
Celery fruit and nut salad	1 pack (250g)	23	418	33
	Per 100g	9	167	13
Chargrilled chicken pasta snack	1 pack (300g)	49	456	21
	Per 100g	16	152	7
Cheese pasta salad	1 pack (200g)	29	504	39
	Per 100g	15	252	20
Cheese, spinach and pine nut pasta salad	1 pack (190g)	75	659	29
	Per 100g	39	347	15
Cherry tomato and rocket pasta	1 pack (225g)	36	223	6
	Per 100g	16	99	2.5
Chicken Caesar salad	1 pack (300g)	32	330	14
	Per 100g	11	110	5
Chicken Caesar pasta salad	1 pack (190g)	45	517	28
	Per 100g	24	272	15
Coleslaw mix	1 pack (440g)	27	136	0.9
	Per 100g	6	31	0.2
Coleslaw salad	1 pack (350g)	15	305	26
	Per 100g	4	87	7
Crayfish, rocket and lemon pasta salad	1 pack (250g)	70	728	40
	Per 100g	28	291	16
Creamy potato salad	1 pack (250g)	30	545	46
	Per 100g	12	218	18

FOOD	SERVING	CARBS (g)	CALS (kcal)	FAT (g)
Crisp mixed salad	1 pack (390g)	12	78	1.2
	Per 100g	3	20	0.3
Fireroast tomato and red pepper pasta salad	1 pack (200g)	38	382	22
	Per 100g	19	191	11
Four leaf salad	1 pack (140g)	2.2	20	0.6
	Per 100g	1.6	14	0.4
Garden salad	1 pack (225g)	5	34	0.7
	Per 100g	2	15	0.3
Green crisp salad	1 pack (180g)	3.1	29	0.9
	Per 100g	1.7	16	0.5
Herb salad	1 pack (100g)	1.8	16	0.5
	Per 100g	1.8	16	0.5
Iceberg lettuce salad	1 pack (300g)	6	39	0.9
	Per 100g	1.9	13	0.3
Italian style salad	1 pack (120g)	2	17	0.6
	Per 100g	1.7	14	0.5
Jardin salad	1 pack (250g)	4	35	1.3
	Per 100g	1.7	14	0.5
Leaf salad	1 pack (115g)	1.7	16	0.5
	Per 100g	1.5	14	0.4
Leafy salad	1 pack (70g)	1.1	10	0.3
	Per 100g	1.5	14	0.4
Mediterranean style bean and smoked tomato salad	1 pack (225g)	28	414	29
	Per 100g	13	184	13
Mediterranean pasta salad	1 pack (350g)	34	305	16
	Per 100g	10	87	5
Moroccan style chicken cous cous salad	1 pack (250g)	46	483	23
	Per 100g	19	193	9
New world salad	1 pack (125g)	0.6	15	0.8
	Per 100g	0.5	12	0.6
Organic crisp mix salad	1 pack (160g)	5	32	0.8
	Per 100g	2.9	20	0.5

Calorie, Fat & Carbohydrate Counter

FOOD	SERVING	CARBS (g)	CALS (kcal)	FAT (g)
Pasta and chargrilled mushrooms	1 pack (200g)	34	404	25
	Per 100g	17	202	13
Potato salad	1 pack (32g)	2	26	2
	Per 100g	8	81	5
Primevera salad	1 pack (100g)	2.4	25	0.6
	Per 100g	2.4	25	0.6
Red cabbage and cranberry slaw	1 pack (250g)	28	150	3.3
	Per 100g	11	60	1.3
Red pepper and coriander cous cous	1 pack (200g)	54	282	3.2
	Per 100g	27	141	1.6
Roast chicken salad	1 pack (300g)	21	348	22
	Per 100g	7	116	7
Rocket salad	1 pack (100g)	0.8	11	0.5
	Per 100g	0.8	11	0.5
Ruby salad	1 pack (170g)	2.7	27	0.7
	Per 100g	1.6	16	0.4
Spicy cous cous	1 pack (250g)	63	325	4
	Per 100g	25	130	1.7
Sundried tomato and chargrilled veg. pasta salad	1 pack (200g)	37	248	8
	Per 100g	19	124	3.9
Sundried tomato and mozzarella pasta	1 pack (225g)	35	394	24
	Per 100g	16	175	11
Sundried tomato potato salad	1 pack (250g)	35	490	37
	Per 100g	14	196	15
Sweet and crunchy salad	1 pack (260g)	8	47	0.8
	Per 100g	3	18	0.3
Sweet shredded salad	1 pack (265g)	8	53	0.5
	Per 100g	2.9	20	0.2
Tabbouleh and feta salad	1 pack (225g)	38	302	11
	Per 100g	17	134	5
Tender leaf salad with mizuna	1 pack (120g)	1.7	18	0.4
	Per 100g	1.4	15	0.3
Tender leaf with mizuna	1 pack (120g)	1.7	18	0.4
	Per 100g	1.4	15	0.3

FOOD	SERVING	CARBS (g)	CALS (kcal)	FAT (g)
Tuna and sweetcorn	1 pack (200g)	34	230	5
	Per 100g	17	115	2.7
Tuna and sweetcorn pasta snack	1 pack (300g)	52	609	37
	Per 100g	17	203	12
Tuna salad	1 pack (370g)	35	466	29
	Per 100g	9	126	8
Waldorf salad	1 pack (250g)	23	455	38
	Per 100g	9	182	15
Watercress salad	1 pack (85g)	0.3	20	0.9
	Per 100g	0.4	23	1
Watercress, spinach and rocket	1 pack (135g)	1.1	30	1.1
	Per 100g	0.8	22	0.8
Wild rocket	1 pack (50g)	0.3	9	0.2
	Per 100g	0.6	18	0.3

Marks & Spencer – salads

FOOD	SERVING	CARBS (g)	CALS (kcal)	FAT (g)
Salads, chicken and smoked bacon	1 pack (380g)	72	817	47
	Per 100g	19	215	12
Salads, honey and mustard chicken	1 pack (380g)	76	741	34
	Per 100g	20	195	9
Salads, king prawns and sun blush	1 pack (100g)	17	225	15
	Per 100g	17	225	15
Salads, noodle salad with sweet chilli and lime chicken	1 pack (380g)	67	570	22
	Per 100g	18	150	6
Salads, Scottish salmon	1 pack (100g)	13	215	15
	Per 100g	13	215	15
Salads, spinach, cheese and pine nuts	1 pack (100g)	16	275	20
	Per 100g	16	275	20
Salads, succulent king prawns and tomatoes	1 pack (380g)	62	366	6
	Per 100g	16	96	1.5
Salads, tomato and basil chicken	1 pack (380g)	63	740	41
	Per 100g	17	195	11

Calorie, Fat & Carbohydrate Counter

FOOD	SERVING	CARBS (g)	CALS (kcal)	FAT (g)
Salads, tuna and sweetcorn pasta salad	1 pack (200g)	37	210	1.8
	Per 100g	18	105	0.9

Sandwiches and wraps

FOOD	SERVING	CARBS (g)	CALS (kcal)	FAT (g)
Chorizo and spicy salsa	1 pack (260g)	75	757	37
	Per 100g	29	291	14
Free range egg and bacon	1 pack (210g)	46	458	20
	Per 100g	22	218	10
Free range egg and tomato	1 pack (165g)	45	314	8
	Per 100g	27	190	5
Ham and cheese	1 pack (206g)	42	548	30
	Per 100g	20	266	15
Mozzarella,tomato and olive	1 pack (256g)	55	904	68
	Per 100g	22	353	27
Pastrami and cheddar cheese	1 pack (261g)	81	679	30
	Per 100g	31	260	12
Pesto and chicken	1 pack (222g)	59	482	14
	Per 100g	26	217	6
Sausage, bacon and egg	1 pack (267g)	53	668	43
	Per 100g	20	250	16
Cheddar with banana chutney	1 pack (217g)	50	584	29
	Per 100g	23	269	13
Extra light soft cheese with oven roasted tomato	1 pack (186g)	45	283	5
	Per 100g	24	152	2.7
Scottish roast beef with horseradish salad	1 pack (200g)	46	546	23
	Per 100g	23	273	12
Smoked turkey with summer salad	1 pack (198g)	44	303	5
	Per 100g	22	153	2.4
York ham and fruit chutney	1 pack (209g)	44	343	9
	Per 100g	21	164	4

Tesco – sandwiches

FOOD	SERVING	CARBS (g)	CALS (kcal)	FAT (g)
All day breakfast sandwich	1 pack (275g)	45	660	42
	Per 100g	16	240	15

FOOD	SERVING	CARBS (g)	CALS (kcal)	FAT (g)
Bagel, B.L.T	1 pack (164g)	63	489	18
	Per 100g	38	298	11
Bagel, chicken caesar	1 pack (184g)	43	392	15
	Per 100g	24	213	8
Bagel, smoked salmon and soft cheese	1 pack (162g)	43	424	18
	Per 100g	27	262	11
Bagel, tuna crunch	1 pack (185g)	44	438	21
	Per 100g	24	237	12
Beef	1 pack (209g)	39	401	17
	Per 100g	19	192	8
Cheese and onion baton	1 pack (212g)	50	655	40
	Per 100g	24	309	19
Cheese and spring onion	1 pack (191g)	34	720	54
	Per 100g	18	377	28
Cheese top roll with ham salad	1 pack (209g)	45	468	24
	Per 100g	22	224	12
Chicken and bacon	1 pack (183g)	45	284	3.1
	Per 100g	25	155	1.7
Chicken and sweetcorn	1 pack (194g)	43	433	21
	Per 100g	22	223	11
Chicken tikka	1 pack (184g)	39	434	20
	Per 100g	21	236	11
Chicken, bacon and avocado	1 pack (209g)	40	518	28
	Per 100g	19	248	14
Chicken, bacon and tomato sandwich	1 pack (211g)	42	502	25
	Per 100g	20	238	12
Ciabatta – lemon and black pepper chicken	1 pack (189g)	46	450	22
	Per 100g	24	238	12
Ciabatta – tuna, olive and basil	1 pack (225g)	44	491	26
	Per 100g	19	218	12
Coriander chicken and mango naan style pocket	1 pack (195g)	50	429	17
	Per 100g	26	220	9
Crayfish and rocket	1 pack (193g)	29	486	31
	Per 100g	15	252	16

Calorie, Fat & Carbohydrate Counter

FOOD	SERVING	CARBS (g)	CALS (kcal)	FAT (g)
Egg salad	1 pack (182g)	36	264	8
	Per 100g	20	145	4
Focaccia – pepperoni, parmesan and rocket	1 pack (199g)	4	659	45
	Per 100g	2.2	331	23
Focaccia – tomato and basil chicken	1 pack (214g)	44	582	36
	Per 100g	20	272	17
Free range egg and bacon	1 pack (199g)	40	519	29
	Per 100g	20	261	14
Free range egg and cress	1 pack (195g)	25	402	24
	Per 100g	13	206	13
Ham and cheese wedge	1 pack (212g)	58	655	37
	Per 100g	27	309	17
Ham egg and tomato baton	1 pack (212g)	49	460	20
	Per 100g	23	217	10
Hot steak sandwich	1 pack (185g)	56	463	19
	Per 100g	30	250	10
Organic cheese and tomato	1 pack (185g)	36	574	36
	Per 100g	20	310	20
Organic egg and tomato	1 pack (185g)	167	387	20
	Per 100g	19	209	11
Ploughmans	1 pack (242g)	45	595	35
	Per 100g	19	246	14
Prawn mayonnaise	1 pack (154g)	18	270	6
	Per 100g	12	175	4
Red cheddar and tomato	1 pack (207g)	44	669	45
	Per 100g	21	323	22
Red salmon and cucumber	1 pack (144g)	35	300	11
	Per 100g	24	208	8
Roast chicken and bacon	1 pack (209g)	40	640	40
	Per 100g	19	306	19
Roast chicken and ham	1 pack (228g)	38	561	32
	Per 100g	17	246	14
Roast chicken and salad	1 pack (224g)	38	435	21
	Per 100g	17	194	10

FOOD	SERVING	CARBS (g)	CALS (kcal)	FAT (g)
Roast chicken and stuffing	1 pack (164g)	40	372	14
	Per 100g	24	227	8
Sausage and egg wedge	1 pack (269g)	63	699	39
	Per 100g	24	260	14
Smoked ham and cheddar	1 pack (204g)	40	620	38
	Per 100g	20	304	19
Smoked ham and mustard	1 pack (159g)	31	417	25
	Per 100g	20	262	16
Smoked ham, soft cheese and pineapple bap	1 pack (202g)	60	339	26
	Per 100g	30	168	13
Smoked salmon and full fat soft cheese	1 pack (200g)	34	450	30
	Per 100g	17	225	15
Tuna and sweetcorn	1 pack (203g)	41	564	33
	Per 100g	18	150	6
Tuna salad	1 pack (197g)	41	427	21
	Per 100g	13	215	15
Chicken and bacon baton	1 pack (201g)	50	511	26
	Per 100g	16	275	20

Tesco – wraps

FOOD	SERVING	CARBS (g)	CALS (kcal)	FAT (g)
Chicken salsa	1 pack (120g)	26	174	3.1
	Per 100g	22	145	2.6
Chicken fajita	1 pack (110g)	27	199	6
	Per 100g	25	181	6
Moroccan style cous cous	1 pack (120g)	33	185	3.1
	Per 100g	27	154	2.6
Chicken caesar	1 pack (103g)	26	236	10
	Per 100g	25	229	10
Bean and cheese	1 pack (105g)	30	258	13
	Per 100g	29	246	12

Marks & Spencer – lunchtime foods

FOOD	SERVING	CARBS (g)	CALS (kcal)	FAT (g)
COU, chilli beef wrap	1 pack (174g)	39	270	3.8
	Per 100g	22	155	2.2

Calorie, Fat & Carbohydrate Counter

FOOD	SERVING	CARBS (g)	CALS (kcal)	FAT (g)
COU, Chinese chicken flatbread	1 pack (155g)	37	240	2.8
	Per 100g	24	155	1.8
COU, ham and cheese pretzel	1 pack (136g)	33	245	3.3
	Per 100g	25	180	2.4
COU, Moroccan style flatbread	1 pack (184g)	56	294	1.5
	Per 100g	31	160	0.8
COU, ranchers chicken flatbread	1 pack (173g)	42	260	3.5
	Per 100g	24	150	2
COU, sandwiches, bacon, lettuce and tomato	1 pack (174g)	39	270	4
	Per 100g	22	155	2.3
COU, sandwiches, chicken and bacon	1 pack (177g)	45	266	3.5
	Per 100g	25	150	2
COU, sandwiches, chicken and salad	1 pack (181g)	36	244	4
	Per 100g	20	135	2.4
COU, sandwiches, chicken caesar	1 pack (193g)	37	261	3.7
	Per 100g	19	135	1.9
COU, sandwiches, lean danish ham and salad	1 pack (188g)	37	244	1.7
	Per 100g	20	130	0.9
COU, sandwiches, roast chicken, no mayo	1 pack (147g)	31	250	3.8
	Per 100g	21	170	2.6
COU, sandwiches, smoked ham and cheese	1 pack (174g)	35	270	3.1
	Per 100g	20	155	1.8
COU, sandwiches, tuna and sweetcorn	1 pack (180g)	40	270	4
	Per 100g	22	150	2.4
Food to Go, all day breakfast	1 pack (196g)	42	529	31
	Per 100g	21	270	16
Food to Go, bacon, lettuce and tomatoes	1 pack (248g)	58	670	38
	Per 100g	23	270	15
Food to Go, chargrilled chicken, pitta bread	1 pack (208g)	30	279	7
	Per 100g	15	134	3.5
Food to Go, chicken and bacon	1 pack (173g)	41	450	21
	Per 100g	24	260	12
Food to Go, chicken and salad	1 pack (193g)	37	261	3.7
	Per 100g	19	135	1.9

FOOD	SERVING	CARBS (g)	CALS (kcal)	FAT (g)
Food to Go, chicken and salad sub	1 pack (238g)	50	571	29
	Per 100g	21	240	12
Food to Go, chicken and stuffing	1 pack (184g)	45	451	24
	Per 100g	24	245	13
Food to Go, chicken caesar salad sub	1 pack (233g)	50	606	32
	Per 100g	21	260	14
food to Go, chicken, bacon and avocado	1 pack (239g)	43	550	30
	Per 100g	18	230	13
Food to Go, chicken and bacon sub	1 pack (218g)	54	545	22
	Per 100g	25	250	10
Food to Go, free range egg and prawn roll	1 pack (200g)	35	530	35
	Per 100g	18	265	17
Food to Go, free range egg and smoked ham	1 pack (200g)	36	480	27
	Per 100g	18	240	14
Food to Go, ham and swiss cheese	1 pack (165g)	31	404	21
	Per 100g	19	245	13
Food to Go, hoisin duck wrap	1 pack (232g)	57	510	22
	Per 100g	24	220	9
Food to Go, Mexican chicken wrap	1 pack (241g)	47	494	25
	Per 100g	20	205	10
Food to Go, poached salmon	1 pack (172g)	28	396	22
	Per 100g	16	230	13
Food to Go, tuna and cucumber	1 pack (171g)	31	436	25
	Per 100g	18	255	15
Food to Go, tuna niçoise wrap	1 pack (281g)	51	660	40
	Per 100g	18	235	14
Salads, chicken and smoked bacon	1 pack (379g)	72	815	47
	Per 100g	19	215	12
Salads, honey and mustard chicken	1 pack (379g)	76	739	34
	Per 100g	20	195	9
Salads, king prawns and sun blush	1 pack (100g)	17	225	15
	Per 100g	17	225	15

Calorie, Fat & Carbohydrate Counter

FOOD	SERVING	CARBS (g)	CALS (kcal)	FAT (g)
Salads, noodle salad with sweet chilli and lime chicken	1 pack (380g)	67	570	22
	Per 100g	18	150	6
Salads, Scottish salmon	1 pack (100g)	13	215	15
	Per 100g	13	215	15
Salads, spinach, cheese and pine nuts	1 pack (100g)	16	275	20
	Per 100g	16	275	20
Salads, succulent king prawns and tomatoes	1 pack (250g)	40	2312	3.8
	Per 100g	16	925	1.5
Salads, tomato and basil chicken	1 pack (379g)	63	739	41
	Per 100g	17	195	11
Salads, tuna and sweetcorn pasta salad	1 pack (200g)	37	210	1.8
	Per 100g	18	105	0.9
Sandwiches, cheddar cheese ploughmans	1 pack (194g)	46	456	24
	Per 100g	24	235	12
Sandwiches, cheese and celery	1 pack (179g)	26	465	31
	Per 100g	15	260	17
Sandwiches, cheese and coleslaw	1 pack (185g)	33	500	32
	Per 100g	18	270	17
Sandwiches, chicken and sweetcorn	1 pack (140g)	28	294	14
	Per 100g	20	210	10
Sandwiches, coronation chicken	1 pack (210g)	42	420	20
	Per 100g	20	200	10
Sandwiches, free range egg and cress	1 pack (180g)	37	270	10
	Per 100g	21	150	6
Sandwiches, free range eggs and bacon	1 pack (257g)	39	655	40
	Per 100g	15	255	16
Sandwiches, tuna salad	1 pack (250g)	42	575	32
	Per 100g	17	230	13
Sandwiches, turkey and ham	1 pack (182g)	31	410	23
	Per 100g	17	225	12
Sandwiches, Wensleydale cheese and carrot	1 pack (183g)	39	430	23
	Per 100g	21	235	12

FOOD	SERVING	CARBS (g)	CALS (kcal)	FAT (g)
Snacks to Go, chargrilled chicken	1 pack (190g)	26	295	15
	Per 100g	14	155	8
Snacks to Go, coronation style chicken salad	1 pack (230g)	53	380	36
	Per 100g	23	165	16
Snacks to Go, feta cheese and tomato	1 pack (189g)	33	359	21
	Per 100g	17	190	11
Snacks to Go, Japanese noodle box, aromatic duck	1 pack (295g)	40	295	6
	Per 100g	13	100	2.1
Snacks to Go, niçoise salad	1 pack (330g)	16	330	22
	Per 100g	5	100	7
Snacks to Go, tapas selection	1 pack (155g)	29	395	23
	Per 100g	18	255	15
Sushi, California roll sushi box	1 pack (230g)	51	391	12
	Per 100g	22	170	5
Sushi, fish selection box	1 pack (220g)	53	396	10
	Per 100g	24	180	5
Sushi, nigiri sushi box	1 pack (190g)	49	285	5
	Per 100g	26	150	2.5
Sushi, sushi to share	1 pack (370g)	81	574	8
	Per 100g	22	155	2.2
Sushi, sushi to snack	1 pack (110g)	27	198	3
	Per 100g	25	180	2.7

5
Cooked meals

Calorie, Fat & Carbohydrate Counter

FOOD	SERVING	CARBS (g)	CALS (kcal)	FAT (g)

PASTA

FOOD	SERVING	CARBS (g)	CALS (kcal)	FAT (g)
Chicken and bacon pasta bake (Tesco)	1 oz (28g)	5	46	1.9
	Per 100g	19	166	7
Chicken and bacon, lasagna (Findus)	1 pack (330g)	37	413	21
	Per 100g	11.3	125	6.2
Chicken and broccoli pasta bake (Weight Watchers)	1 pack (305g)	43	290	5
	Per 100g	14	95	1.5
Chicken and pasta gratin (Somerfield)	1 pack (500g)	45	825	55
	Per 100g	9	165	11
Fusilli, BGTY (Sainsbury's)	1 pack (400g)	34	304	8
	Per 100g	8.6	76	2
Lasagna creamy pasta bake (Napolina)	1 jar (525g)	49	452	21
	Per 100g	9.4	86	4
Lasagna pies (Farmfoods)	1 pie (269g)	39	341	16
	Per 100g	23	202	9.3
Lasagna (Bird's Eye)	1 meal (375g)	43	420	17
	Per 100g	12	112	4.6
Lasagna, COU (Marks & Spencer)	1 pack (300g)	38	285	7
	Per 100g	12.8	95	2.2
Lasagna (Linda McCartney)	1 pack (320g)	45	374	11
	Per 100g	14	117	3.5
Lasagna, ready meals (Marks & Spencer)	1 pack (360g)	42	594	30
	Per 100g	12	165	8.2
Lasagna, vegetable, average	1 oz (28g)	3.5	29	1.2
	Per 100g	12.4	102	4.4
Macaroni Bolognaise (Somerfield)	1 pack (500g)	100	760	30
	Per 100g	30	152	6
Macaroni cheese, Pasta n' Sauce (Batchelor's)	1 pack (115g)	73	435	7
	Per 100g	64	378	6
Pasat Pronto, mushroom and garlic (Safeway)	1 pack (203g)	44	315	11
	Per 100g	22	155	5.3
Pasta arrabiata (Tesco)	1 pack (205g)	25	144	2.5
	Per 100g	12	70	1.2

FOOD	SERVING	CARBS (g)	CALS (kcal)	FAT (g)
Pasta bake, pepperoni (Dolmio)	1 pack (250g)	25	215	9
	Per 100g	9	86	3.9
Pasta Bolognaise, chilled (Co-op)	1 pack (300g)	57	345	6
	Per 100g	19	115	2
Pasta Fasta, bolognaise (Ross)	1 pack (300g)	48	270	1.8
	Per 100g	16	90	0.6
Pasta fungi with croutons, Taste breaks (Knorr)	1 pack (350g)	59	424	16
	Per 100g	17	121	4.6
Spaghetti and meat balls (Somerfield)	1 pack (350g)	53	403	14
	Per 100g	15	115	4
Spaghetti and vegetarian meatballs (Safeway)	1 pack (350g)	48	382	13
	Per 100g	14	109	3.8
Spaghetti bolognaise (Sainsbury's)	1 pack (300g)	31	237	6
	Per 100g	11	39	1.9
Spaghetti bolognaise, average	1 oz (28g)	23	96	0
	Per 100g	81	341	0.01
Spaghetti bolognaise (Bird's Eye)	1 pack (362g)	48	404	16
	Per 100g	13	112	4.4
Spaghetti bolognaise, Healthy Choice (Iceland)	1 pack (400g)	71	428	4
	Per 100g	17	107	1
Spaghetti carbonara (Somerfield)	1 pack (300g)	39	501	33
	Per 100g	13	167	11
Tagliatelle carbonara, Low fat (Bertorelli)	1 pack (350g)	42	301	8
	Per 100g	12	86	2.2
Tagliatelle carbonara, Ready Meals (Waitrose)	1 pack (350g)	35	749	57
	Per 100g	10	214	16
Tagliatelle carbonara, Reduced fat (Waitrose)	1 pack (350g)	42	399	18
	Per 100g	12	114	5.1
Tagliatelle niçoise (Waitrose)	1 pack (500g)	70	785	49
	Per 100g	14	157	9.8
Tagliatelle with chicken, garlic and lemon, BGTY (Sainsbury's)	1 pack (450g)	49	509	17
	Per 100g	11	113	3.8

Calorie, Fat & Carbohydrate Counter

FOOD	SERVING	CARBS (g)	CALS (kcal)	FAT (g)
Tuna and pasta bake (Co-op)	1 pack (340g)	44	371	11
	Per 100g	13	109	3.3
Tuna and pasta bake (Somerfield)	1 pack (300g)	30	411	21
	Per 100g	10	137	7
Tuna creamy pasta bake (Napolina)	1 jar (525g)	60	488	20
	Per 100g	12	93	8.8

FOOD	SERVING	CARBS (g)	CALS (kcal)	FAT (g)

PIZZA

FOOD	SERVING	CARBS (g)	CALS (kcal)	FAT (g)
Cheese and tomato pizza, 9.5 inch (Domino)	1 slice (52g)	18	125	2.9
	Per 100g	35	241	5.6
Cheese and tomato pizza, Deep and Crispy (Tesco)	1 slice (45g)	9	65	1.9
	Per 100g	32	231	6.8
Cheese and tomato pizza, Thin and Crispy (Morrisons)	1 pizza (335g)	92	787	29
	Per 100g	27	235	8.7
Ham and mushroom pizza, cooked, Freschetta (Schwan's)	1 pizza (360g)	107	860	28
	Per 100g	30	239	7.8
Ham and mushroom pizza, COU (Marks & Spencer)	1 pack (245g)	63	392	6
	Per 100g	26	160	2.4
Ham and mushroom pizza, Deep Dish (Schwan's)	1 pizza (170g)	50	383	13
	Per 100g	30	225	7.5
Ham and mushroom pizza, Thin and Crispy (Marks & Spencer)	1 pizza (340g)	87	680	25
	Per 100g	26	200	7.2
Ham and pineapple pizza (Chicago Town)	1 pizza (435g)	129	866	20
	Per 100g	30	199	4.5
Ham and pineapple pizza, stonebaked (Marks & Spencer)	1 pizza (345g)	98	690	20
	Per 100g	28	200	5.7
Pepperoni pizza, American style Deep Pan (Co-op)	1 pizza (305g)	110	988	40
	Per 100g	28	250	10
Pepperoni pizza, Deep and Crispy (Tesco)	1 pizza (375g)	120	881	28
	Per 100g	32	235	7.5
Pepperoni pizza, Italian, Thin and Crispy (Morrisons)	1 pizza (365g)	91	843	35
	Per 100g	25	231	9.6

Calorie, Fat & Carbohydrate Counter

FOOD	SERVING	CARBS (g)	CALS (kcal)	FAT (g)
Pizza base, stonebaked (Napolina)	1 base (75g)	99	474	2.6
	Per 100g	58	279	1.5
Pizza base, Thin and Crispy (Napolina)	1 base (150g)	87	437	5
	Per 100g	58	291	3
Pizza, cheese and tomato, average	1 slice (45g)	11	107	3.6
	Per 100g	25	237	8
Pizza, tomato, average	1 slice (45g)	10	87	3.2
	Per 100g	22	193	7
Spinach and ricotta pizza, Classico (Tesco)	1 pizza (208g)	57	437	15
	Per 100g	27	210	7.3
Spinach and ricotta pizza, Pizzeroma (Safeway)	1 pizza (420g)	132	1042	37
	Per 100g	31	248	8.8

FOOD	SERVING	CARBS (g)	CALS (kcal)	FAT (g)

INDIAN

FOOD	SERVING	CARBS (g)	CALS (kcal)	FAT (g)
Chicken and rice (Iceland)	1 pack (400g)	54	455	30
	Per 100g	14	114	3.3
Chicken Balti and rice (Pataks)	1 pack (370g)	620	440	13
	Per 100g	17	119	3.5
Chicken Balti with naan bread (Sharwoods)	1 pack (375g)	58	540	24
	Per 100g	15	144	6.3
Chicken Balti with rice (Weight Watchers)	1 serving (329g)	35	253	6
	Per 100g	11	77	1.7
Chicken Balti, COU (Marks & Spencer)	1 pack (400g)	54	360	3.6
	Per 100g	14	90	0.9
Chicken Balti, Snap pot (Pataks)	1 snack pot (220g)	28	202	6
	Per 100g	13	92	2.8
Chicken Biryani (Somerfield)	1 pack (300g)	57	477	18
	Per 100g	20	159	6
Chicken curry and potato wedges, Healthy Eating (Tesco)	1 pack (450g)	45	428	12
	Per 100g	10	95	2.7
Chicken curry and potato (Marks & Spencer)	1 oz (28g)	4	53	3.2
	Per 100g	15	190	12
Chicken curry with chips (Bird's Eye)	1 pack (380g)	78	475	8
	Per 100g	21	125	2.2
Chicken curry, extra strong (Marks & Spencer)	1 oz (28g)	0.7	28	1.1
	Per 100g	2.5	100	4
Chicken curry (Pot Rice)	1 pot (74g)	50	253	1.7
	Per 100g	67	342	2.3
Chicken Jalfrezi with basmati rice, frozen (Co-op)	1 pack (340g)	48	391	14
	Per 100g	14	115	4
Chicken Jalfrezi with mustard seed rice (Somerfield)	1 pack (340g)	58	428	14
	Per 100g	17	126	4

Calorie, Fat & Carbohydrate Counter

FOOD	SERVING	CARBS (g)	CALS (kcal)	FAT (g)
Chicken Jalfrezi with pilau rice, BGTY (Sainsbury's)	1 pack (450g)	64	432	5
	Per 100g	14	96	1.2
Chicken Jalfrezi wrap (Pataks)	1 wrap (150g)	32	264	12
	Per 100g	21	176	8
Chicken Jalfrezi (Safeway)	1 pack (333g)	15	360	15
	Per 100g	4.5	108	4.6
Chicken Korma and pilau rice, BGTY (Sainsbury's)	1 meal (450g)	66	513	10
	Per 100g	15	114	2.2
Chicken Korma and rice (Pataks)	1 pack (370g)	59	466	18
	Per 100g	16	126	4.8
Chicken mMadras with pilau rice (Eastern Classics)	1 pack (400g)	59	616	29
	Per 100g	15	154	7.2
Chicken Madras (Tesco)	1 meal (350g)	13	326	14
	Per 100g	3.6	93	4.1
Chicken Tikka Masala and basmati rice (Pataks)	1 pack (400g)	60	580	20
	Per 100g	15	145	5
Chicken Tikka Biriani with basmati rice (Sharwoods)	1 pack (373g)	60	481	16
	Per 100g	16	129	4.3
Lamb curry with rice (Bird's Eye)	1 pack (382g)	80	520	13
	Per 100g	21	136	3.4
Lamb curry, extra strong (Marks & Spencer)	1 oz (28g)	1.3	35	1.9
	Per 100g	4.6	125	6.9
Lamb samosa (Waitrose)	1 oz (28g)	5	87	6
	Per 100g	18	310	23
Prawn Bhuna, Indian Tandoori (Sainsbury's)	Half pack (200g)	9	152	8
	Per 100g	4.5	76	4
Prawn curry with rice (Bird's Eye)	1 pack (381g)	78	450	9
	Per 100g	21	118	2.4
Prawn Rogan Josh, COU (Marks & Spencer)	1 serving (400g)	65	360	2.4
	Per 100g	16	90	0.6

FOOD	SERVING	CARBS (g)	CALS (kcal)	FAT (g)
CHINESE				
Chicken & black bean noodles (Sainsbury's)	1 pack (350g)	84	417	2.5
	Per 100g	24	119	0.7
Chicken & black bean sauce & egg rice, HE (Tesco)	1 pack (400g)	50	372	9
	Per 100g	12	93	2.3
Chicken & cashew nuts & veg rice, COU (Marks & Spencer)	1 pack (400g)	34	320	8
	Per 100g	9	80	2
Chicken & cashew nuts with egg fried rice (Somerfield)	1 pack (340g)	44	435	17
	Per 100g	13	128	5
Chicken & mushroom with egg fried rice (Farmfoods)	1 meal (325g)	49	374	12
	Per 100g	15	115	4
Chicken & pineapple with egg fried rice (Tesco)	1 pack (450g)	55	450	11
	Per 100g	12	100	2.4
Chicken chow mein (Co-Op)	1 pack (300g)	27	270	9
	Per 100g	9	90	3
Chicken chow mein, HE (Tesco)	1 pack (450g)	49	392	5
	Per 100g	11	87	1.2
Chicken in black bean sauce with egg fried rice (Somerfield)	1 pack (340g)	44	384	14
	Per 100g	13	113	4
Chicken in black bean sauce with rice (Iceland)	1 pack (400g)	63	388	6
	Per 100g	16	97	1.5
Chow Mein (Vesta)	1 meal (107g)	58	340	5
	Per 100g	54	318	4.7
Chow Mein Pot Noodle (Pot Noodle)	1 pot 89g	54	385	14
	Per 100g	61	433	16
Chow Mein, Ready meals (Waitrose)	1 pack (450g)	37	365	21
	Per 100g	8	81	4.6
Chow Mein stir fry (Asda)	1 pack (350g)	21	270	18
	Per 100g	6	77	5

Calorie, Fat & Carbohydrate Counter

FOOD	SERVING	CARBS (g)	CALS (kcal)	FAT (g)
Pork stir fry, HE (Tesco)	1 serving (150g)	0	152	2.4
	Per 100g	0	101	1.6
Prawn & Chinese greens (Marks & Spencer)	1 pack (300g)	14	180	7
	Per 100g	4.8	60	2.3
Prawn crackers (Sainsbury's)	1 cracker (3g)	1.8	16	1
	Per 100g	60	537	32
Prawn crackers, uncooked (Sharwoods)	1 cracker (3g)	1.6	15	0.9
	Per 100g	53	487	30
Seaweed (Wakame) dried, raw	28g	0	38	0.4
	Per 100g	0	136	1.5
Spare ribs (Marks & Spencer)	28g	2.4	57	3.2
	Per 100g	9	205	12
Spare ribs sweet Chinese style (Co-Op)	1 pack (250g)	40	553	28
	Per 100g	16	221	11
Special Chinese curry with egg fried rice (Farmfoods)	1 pack (325g)	57	452	17
	Per 100g	18	139	5
Special Chow Mein (Mayflower)	1 pack (340g)	21	323	15
	Per 100g	6	95	4.4
Special fried rice (Marks & Spencer)	1 serving (100g)	27	205	8
	Per 100g	27	205	8
Spring rolls (Co-Op)	28g	8	67	3.1
	Per 100g	29	240	11
Sweet & sour chicken, HC (Safeway)	1 pack (400g)	102	580	7.2
	Per 100g	26	145	1.8
Sweet & sour chicken (Weight Watchers)	1 pack (320g)	56	304	1.3
	Per 100g	17	95	0.4
Sweet & sour chicken rice bowl (Sharwoods)	1 bowl (350g)	65	438	12
	Per 100g	19	125	3.5
Sweet & sour chicken with rice (Oriental Express)	1 pack (340g)	72	350	2
	Per 100g	21	103	0.6

FOOD	SERVING	CARBS (g)	CALS (kcal)	FAT (g)
Sweet & sour pork, Ready Meals (Marks & Spencer)	28g	6	48	1.7
	Per 100g	22	170	6
Sweet & sour Pot Noodle (Pot Noodle)	1 pot (86g)	54	376	14
	Per 100g	63	437	16

Calorie, Fat & Carbohydrate Counter

FOOD	SERVING	CARBS (g)	CALS (kcal)	FAT (g)

THAI

FOOD	SERVING	CARBS (g)	CALS (kcal)	FAT (g)
Thai Chiang Mai chicken & noodles, BGTY (Sainsbury's)	1 pack 448g	49	484	18
	Per 100g	11	108	4
Thai chicken & lemongrass (Batchelor's)	1 sachet 278g	15	127	6.6
	Per 100g	5	46	2.4
Thai chicken (Bird's Eye)	1 portion 86g	2.7	189	13
	Per 100g	3.1	220	15
Thai chicken curry tom yum (Sainsbury's)	1 pot 400g	14	416	20
	Per 100g	3.5	104	5.1
Thai coconut chicken & noodles (M&S)	1 pack 400g	32	320	7
	Per 100g	8	80	1.8
Thai curry Supernoodles (Batchelor's)	1 serving 290g	63	481	63
	Per 100g	22	166	8
Thai fragrant mussels (M&S)	1/2 pack 325g	15	358	19
	Per 100g	4.5	110	5.7
Thai green curry mini fillets (Sainsbury's)	1/2 pack 100g	0.9	130	1.6
	Per 100g	0.9	130	1.6
Thai green curry, Ready Meals (M&S)	1 pack 300g	6	375	25
	Per 100g	2	125	8
Thai prawns (M&S)	28g	3.8	29	0.9
	Per 100g	14	103	3.1
Thai red chicken curry (Asda)	1 pack 360g	20	461	28
	Per 100g	6	128	8
Thai red chicken curry, BGTY (Sainsbury's)	1 pack 450g	67	545	19
	Per 100g	15	121	4.1
Thai red chicken curry with fragrant rice (Somerfield)	1 pack 340g	61	503	17
	Per 100g	18	148	5
Thai style chicken, BGTY (Sainsbury's)	1 serving 190g	13	247	9
	Per 100g	7	130	4.5
Thai style fish cakes (Sainsbury's)	1 fish cake 49g	7	69	2.1
	Per 100g	14	141	4.2

FOOD	SERVING	CARBS (g)	CALS (kcal)	FAT (g)
QUICHES				
Broccoli & tomato quiche Reduced Fat (Somerfield)	1 quiche (325g)	88	839	42
	Per 100g	27	258	13
Broccoli, tomato & cheese quiche BGTY (Sainsbury's)	1 quiche (390g)	61	632	32
	Per 100g	16	162	8.2
Cheese & bacon quiche, Healthy Eating (Tesco)	1 serving (155g)	31	307	14
	Per 100g	20	198	9
Cheese & bacon quiche, Smart Price (Asda)	1/4 quiche (82g)	16	208	14
	Per 100g	20	257	17
Cheese & broccoli quiche, Good Intentions (Somerfield)	1 quiche (145g)	26	229	13
	Per 100g	18	158	9
Cheese & ham quiche (Somerfield)	1 quiche (325g)	59	835	59
	Per 100g	18	257	18
Cheese & onion quiche (Sainsbury's)	1 quiche (390g)	59	956	66
	Per 100g	15	245	17
Cheese & onion quiche (Somerfield)	1 quiche (300g)	42	696	48
	Per 100g	14	232	16
Cheese & tomato quiche 4 (Somerfield)	1 quiche (135g)	31	416	26
	Per 100g	23	308	19
Cheese & tomato quiche (Morrison)	1/2 quiche (64g)	14	195	13
	Per 100g	23	304	21
Cheese onion & chive quiche (Somerfield)	1 sm quiche (110g)	19	326	24
	Per 100g	17	296	22
Cheese potato & onion quiche (Safeway)	1/3 quiche (115g)	28	361	23
	Per 100g	24	314	20
Mediterranean vegetable quiche, BGTY (Sainsbury's)	1 serving (100g)	34	392	22
	Per 100g	34	392	22
Mediterranean vegetable quiche (Sainsbury's)	1/3 quiche (133g)	19	321	23
	Per 100g	15	241	18

Calorie, Fat & Carbohydrate Counter

FOOD	SERVING	CARBS (g)	CALS (kcal)	FAT (g)
Mushroom quiche (Morrisons)	1/4 quiche (85g)	15	241	17
	Per 100g	18	283	19
Mushroom quiche (Safeway)	1/4 quiche (82g)	15	192	12
	Per 100g	18	234	15
Spinach & ricotta quiche (Safeway)	1/4 quiche (85g)	19	193	10
	Per 100g	23	227	12
Spinach, ricotta & gruyere quiche slice (Somerfield)	1 slice (130g)	20	348	26
	Per 100g	15	268	20

FOOD	SERVING	CARBS (g)	CALS (kcal)	FAT (g)
OTHER MEAT DISHES				
Beef steak pudding	1 Serving (250g)	45	588	30
	Per 100g	18	235	12
Beef stew	1 Serving (250g)	13	300	18
	Per 100g	5	120	7
Chilli con carne	1 Serving (250g)	20	388	23
	Per 100g	8	155	9
Hot pot	1 Serving (250g)	25	288	13
	Per 100g	10	115	5
Irish stew	1 Serving (250g)	23	313	20
	Per 100g	9	125	8
Lamb keema	1 Serving (250g)	6	850	75
	Per 100g	2.4	340	30
Moussaka	1 Serving (250g)	18	475	35
	Per 100g	7	190	14
Pancake roll	1 Serving (250g)	55	575	33
	Per 100g	22	230	13
Shepherd's pie	1 Serving (250g)	20	300	15
	Per 100g	8	120	6
Black pudding, fried	1 serving (120g)	18	378	26
	Per 100g	15	315	22
Cornish pasty	1 serving (150g)	45	495	30
	Per 100g	30	330	20
Pork pie	1 serving (70g)	18	270	18
	Per 100g	25	385	26
Sausage roll	1 average (50g)	19	223	16
	Per 100g	37	445	32
Sausages, beef, fried	1 average (50g)	8	133	9
	Per 100g	15	265	18
Sausages, beef, grilled	1 average (50g)	7	128	9
	Per 100g	14	255	18
Sausages, pork, fried	1 average (50g)	6	13	
	Per 100g	11	26	0

Calorie, Fat & Carbohydrate Counter

FOOD	SERVING	CARBS (g)	CALS (kcal)	FAT (g)
Sausages, pork, grilled	1 average (50g)	6	158	12
	Per 100g	12	315	24
Sausages, low fat, fried	1 average (50g)	5	108	7
	Per 100g	9	215	13
Sausages, low fat, grilled	1 average (50g)	6	120	7
	Per 100g	11	240	14
Saveloy	1 serving (70g)	7	186	15
	Per 100g	10	265	21
Steak and kidney pie, individual	1 serving (150g)	38	465	30
	Per 100g	25	310	20
Steak and kidney pie, pastry	1 serving (150g)	24	413	26
	Per 100g	16	275	17
Stewed steak, canned with gravy	1 serving (50g)	0.5	93	6
	Per 100g	1	185	12
Haggis, boiled	1 serving (150g)	30	450	32
	Per 100g	20	300	21
White pudding	1 serving (120g)	43	546	38
	Per 100g	36	455	32

FOOD	SERVING	CARBS (g)	CALS (kcal)	FAT (g)
FROZEN FOODS				
Beef Grillsteaks (Bird's Eye)	1 grillsteak (66g)	2.4	205	17
	Per 100g	3.6	307	26
Beef Quarter Pounders (Bird's Eye)	1 burger (139g)	5	386	31
	Per 100g	3.5	278	22
Chicken Burger (Bird's Eye)	1 burger (172g)	30	444	30
	Per 100g	17	258	15
Chicken O's (Bird's Eye)	10 O's (50g)	7	128	8
	Per 100g	14	256	16
Chicken Quarter Pounders (Bird's Eye)	1 burger (117g)	18	280	16
	Per 100g	15	239	14
Chicksticks (Bird's Eye)	3 chicksticks	11	200	13
	Per 100g	15	263	17
Crispy Chicken Dippers (Bird's Eye)	5 grilled	11	210	13
	Per 100g	12	225	14
Crispy Chicken (Bird's Eye)	1 baked	13	230	13
	Per 100g	13	233	13
Crispy Vegetable Fingers (Bird's Eye)	1 finger (10g)	2.1	17	0.8
	Per 100g	21	170	8
Crunchy Garlic Chicken (Bird's Eye)	1 piece (100g)	17	259	15
	Per 100g	17	259	15
Garlic Chargrills (Bird's Eye)	Per chargrill	1.1	170	11
	Per 100g	1.2	222	16
Lamb Grillsteaks (Bird's Eye)	1 (140g)	2.7	335	26
	Per 100g	1.9	239	18
Lamb Quarter Pounders (Bird's Eye)	1 burger (112g)	4.3	232	17
	Per 100g	3.8	207	15
Mega Burgers (Bird's Eye)	Per burger	3	280	21
	Per 100g	2.4	276	22
Mighty Beef Grillsteaks (Bird's Eye)	Per grillsteak	4.4	380	28
	Per 100g	2.3	264	21
Original Chargrills (Bird's Eye)	Per chargrill	1	180	12
	Per 100g	1.1	227	17

Calorie, Fat & Carbohydrate Counter

FOOD	SERVING	CARBS (g)	CALS (kcal)	FAT (g)
Original Vegetable Rice (Bird's Eye)	30g	5.8	29	0.2
	Per 100g	19	96	0.7
Original & Best Beef Burger (Bird's Eye)	Per burger	2	115	8
	Per 100g	3.5	278	23
Pork Quarter Pounders (Bird's Eye)	1/4 pound	3.5	195	15
	Per 100g	3.2	235	22
Vegetable Quarter Pounders (Bird's Eye)	1 burger (100g)	20	166	8
	Per 100g	20	166	8

Chips and potatoes

FOOD	SERVING	CARBS (g)	CALS (kcal)	FAT (g)
Alphabites (Bird's Eye)	9 bites (56g)	11	75	3
	Per 100g	20	134	5
Crispy Potato Fritters (Bird's Eye)	1 fritter (20g)	3.3	29	1.6
	Per 100g	17	145	8
Fish & Chips (Somerfield)	1 serving (250g)	53	420	23
	Per 100g	21	168	9
Hash Browns, deep fried in vegetable oil (McCain)	1 serving (50g)	15	123	8
	Per 100g	31	246	15
Hash Browns, oven baked product (McCain)	1 serving (50g)	15	98	4.5
	Per 100g	30	196	9
House of Horror, deep fried in vegetable oil (McCain)	1 oz (28g)	9	62	2.6
	Per 100g	32	222	9
House of Horror, oven baked product (McCain)	1 oz (28g)	9	62	3
	Per 100g	32	222	9
New Crinkle Cut Oven Chips, (Co-op)	1 serving (100g)	23	146	4
	Per 100g	23	146	4
Potato Smiles, deep fried in vegetable oil (McCain)	1 oz (28g)	9	64	2.7
	Per 100g	32	227	10
Potato Smiles, oven baked product (McCain)	1 oz (28g)	9	62	2.4
	Per 100g	28	192	7

FOOD	SERVING	CARBS (g)	CALS (kcal)	FAT (g)
Potato Speedsters, deep fried in vegetable oil (McCain)	1 oz (28g)	8	60	3
	Per 100g	30	216	9
Potato Waffles (Bird's Eye)	1 waffle (56g)	12	94	4.8
	Per 100g	21	167	9

Fish

FOOD	SERVING	CARBS (g)	CALS (kcal)	FAT (g)
Big Time Cod Cakes (Bird's Eye)	1 cake (114g)	19	185	8
	Per 100g	17	162	7
Breaded Haddock Portions (Somerfield)	1 portion (100g)	13	212	12
	Per 100g	13	212	12
Breaded Whitefish Portions (Somerfield)	1 portion (100g)	13	204	12
	Per 100g	13	204	12
Captain's Cod Pie (Bird's Eye)	1 meal (358g)	36	455	26
	Per 100g	10	127	7
Captain's Coins (Bird's Eye)	1 coin (20g)	2.7	34	1.7
	Per 100g	13	168	8
Chunky Cod Fillets BGTY (Sainsbury's)	1 fillet (139g)	18	228	8
	Per 100g	13	165	5
Cod Fillet Fish Fingers (Bird's Eye)	1 finger (30g)	4.2	53	2.3
	Per 100g	14	194	8
Cod Portions (Somerfield)	1 portion (92g)	0	70	0.9
	Per 100g	0	76	1
Cod Steaks in Butter Sauce (Bird's Eye)	1 pack (170g)	7	165	8
	Per 100g	4	97	5
Cod Steaks in Cheese Sauce (Bird's Eye)	1 pack (182g)	10	175	6
	Per 100g	5	96	4
Cod Steaks in Crispy Batter (Bird's Eye)	1 steak (124g)	14	241	15
	Per 100g	11	194	12
Cod Steaks in Crunch Crumbs (Bird's Eye)	1 steak (103g)	12	224	14
	Per 100g	12	217	13
Cod Steaks in Mushroom Sauce (Bird's Eye)	1 pack (181g)	9	179	8
	Per 100g	5	99	4

Calorie, Fat & Carbohydrate Counter

FOOD	SERVING	CARBS (g)	CALS (kcal)	FAT (g)
Cod Steaks in Parsley Sauce (Bird's Eye)	1 pack (176g)	9	150	4.6
	Per 100g	5	85	3
Fish Cakes (Somerfield)	1 fish cake (42g)	8	75	3.4
	Per 100g	19	178	8
Fish Cakes battered (Farmfoods)	1 fish cake (50g)	38	106	5.5
	Per 100g	19	211	11
Fish Cakes (Bird's Eye)	1 fish cake (52g)	8	89	3.8
	Per 100g	15	172	7
Fish Cakes Mini Captain's Coins (Bird's Eye)	1 fish cake (20g)	2.7	34	1.7
	Per 100g	13	168	8
Fish Choice Fish Steaks in Butter Sauce (Ross)	1 serving (150g)	4.8	126	6
	Per 100g	3.2	84	3.9
Fish Choice Fish Steaks in Parsley Sauce (Ross)	1 serving (150g)	4.7	123	6
	Per 100g	3.1	82	3.7
Fish Fingers in Crispy Batter (Bird's Eye)	1 fish finger (29g)	4.6	63	3.7
	Per 100g	16	218	13
Fish Fingers (Bird's Eye)	1 fish finger (28g)	3.9	50	2.2
	Per 100g	14	177	8
Fish Fingers (Iceland)	1 fish finger (23g)	4	44	2
	Per 100g	17	192	9
Fish in Pastry – Cheese (Bird's Eye)	1 piece (171g)	29	390	23
	Per 100g	17	228	14
Fish & Chips (Safeway)	1 pack (249g)	62	518	21
	Per 100g	25	208	8
Haddock Fillet Fish Fingers (Bird's Eye)	1 finger (29g)	3.8	48	2.1
	Per 100g	13	167	7
Haddock Steaks in Batter, (Marks & Spencer)	1 steak (approx 140g)	3.9	57	3.2
	Per 100g	14	204	12
Haddock Steaks in Breadcrumbs (Marks & Spencer)	1 steak (approx 140g)	3.4	56	2.9
	Per 100g	13	199	10
Haddock Steaks in Crispy Batter (Bird's Eye)	1 steak (145g)	20	307	18
	Per 100g	14	212	13

FOOD	SERVING	CARBS (g)	CALS (kcal)	FAT (g)
Haddock Steaks in Crunch Crumbs (Bird's Eye)	1 steak (103g)	12	224	14
	Per 100g	12	217	13
Pacific Salmon Fillets Lime & Coriander Marinade (Sainsbury's)	1 serving (100g)	1.3	139	4.1
	Per 100g	1.3	139	4.1
Peeled Prawns (Young's)	1 oz (28g)	0	28	0.3
	Per 100g	0	99	0.9
Salmon & Broccoli Pie (Bird's Eye)	1 pie (351g)	40	449	22
	Per 100g	11	128	6
Scottish Island Cocktail Scampi (Youngs)	1 oz (28g)	4.4	50	2.4
	Per 100g	16	179	9
Simply Fish in Crispy Batter (Bird's Eye)	1 steak (120g)	14	230	12
	Per 100g	12	192	10
Skinless Boned Cod in Crispy Batter (Somerfield)	1 portion (150g)	23	303	15
	Per 100g	15	202	10
Smoked Haddock Fillets (Somerfield)	1 serving (130g)	0	105	1.3
	Per 100g	0	81	1
Smoked Haddock Fillets in a Cheese & Chive Sauce (Seafresh)	1 serving (170g)	2	201	10
	Per 100g	1.2	118	6.1
Smoked Haddock in Rich Mustard Sauce (Somerfield)	1 pack (350g)	11	319	11
	Per 100g	3	91	3
Tiger Prawns Cooked & Peeled (Somerfield)	1 pack (180g)	0	122	1.8
	Per 100g	0	68	1

6
Sweets and desserts

FOOD	SERVING	CARBS (g)	CALS (kcal)	FAT (g)
BISCUITS				
Biscuits non-branded (average)				
Chocolate chip	5 (about 60g)	37	247	11
	Per 100g	65	436	19
Coconut bars	5 (about 45g)	29	222	11
	Per 100g	68	522	26
Fig bars	4 (about 60g)	42	200	3.1
	Per 100g	74	353	5
Gingersnaps	5 (about 35g)	28	147	3.1
	Per 100g	79	415	9
Lady fingers	4 (about 45g)	28	158	3.4
	Per 100g	67	372	8
Macaroons	2 (about 45g)	25	181	9
	Per 100g	59	426	21
Marshmallow w/ coconut	4 (about 70g)	52	294	10
	Per 100g	74	415	13
Molasses	2 (about 60g)	49	274	7
	Per 100g	87	483	12
Oatmeal with raisins	4 (about 60g)	38	235	8
	Per 100g	67	414	14
Peanut butter sandwich	4 (about 50g)	33	232	9
	Per 100g	66	468	19
Peanut butter	4 (about 50g)	28	245	14
	Per 100g	56	494	28
Sandwich cookies, chocolate	4 ovals (about 60g)	42	297	14
	Per 100g	73	524	24
Sandwich cookies, vanilla	4 ovals (about 60g)	42	297	14
	Per 100g	73	524	24
Shortbread	5 (about 35g)	24	187	9
	Per 100g	69	528	25
Sugar wafers	5 (about 35g)	35	230	9
	Per 100g	98	649	26

FOOD	SERVING	CARBS (g)	CALS (kcal)	FAT (g)
Sugar, homemade	5 (about 45g)	27	170	6
	Per 100g	63	400	14
Vanilla wafers	10 (about 45g)	30	185	6
	Per 100g	70	435	15

Savoury biscuits

FOOD	SERVING	CARBS (g)	CALS (kcal)	FAT (g)
Bath Oliver, large (Jacob's)	1 biscuit (12g)	8	52	1.6
	Per 100g	67	435	15
Cheddars (McVitie's)	1 biscuit (4g)	2.2	22	1.3
	Per 100g	50	540	31
Cheese Melts (Carr's)	1 biscuit (4g)	2.6	21	1
	Per 100g	58	468	22
Choicegrain Crackers (Jacob's)	1 biscuit (7g)	5	32	1.1
	Per 100g	65	435	15
Crackerbread (Ryvita)	1 biscuit (5g)	4	19	0.2
	Per 100g	79	383	3
Cream Crackers	1 biscuit (8g)	6	35	1.1
	Per 100g	70	440	15
Hovis Cracker (Jacob's)	1 biscuit (6g)	3.7	27	1.1
	Per 100g	62	454	19
Krackawheat (McVitie's)	1 biscuit (7g)	5	38	2
	Per 100g	62	515	25
Matzo Crackers (Rakusen)	1 biscuit (4g)	3.2	15	0.1
	Per 100g	84	367	2
Melts (Carr's)	1 biscuit (4g)	2.3	19	0.9
	Per 100g	58	451	20
Mini Ritz Crackers (Jacob's)	1 biscuit (3g)	1.8	17	1
	Per 100g	56	534	32
Original Ryvita	1 biscuit (9g)	0.5	2.4	0
	Per 100g	6	27	0
Sesame Ryvita	1 biscuit (9g)	0.5	2.8	0.1
	Per 100g	5	31	1
Table Water Biscuits, large (Carr's)	1 biscuit (7g)	6	33	0.7
	Per 100g	77	441	9

Calorie, Fat & Carbohydrate Counter

FOOD	SERVING	CARBS (g)	CALS (kcal)	FAT (g)
Table Water Biscuits, small (Carr's)	1 biscuit (3g)	2.6	15	0.3
	Per 100g	77	445	9
Tuc Biscuits (McVitie's)	1 biscuit (5g)	2.7	25	1.3
	Per 100g	58	533	28

Sweet biscuits

FOOD	SERVING	CARBS (g)	CALS (kcal)	FAT (g)
Abbey Crunch (McVitie's)	1 biscuit (10g)	7	46	1.7
	Per 100g	73	479	18
Ace – Milk Chocolate (McVitie's)	1 biscuit (25g)	17	125	6
	Per 100g	68	510	25
All Butter Shortbread (McVitie's)	1 biscuit (14g)	4	77	4
	Per 100g	30	541	30
Animal Biscuits (Cadbury's)	1 biscuit (25g)	18	125	5
	Per 100g	70	493	21
Blue Riband (Nestlé)	1 biscuit (21g)	14	109	6
	Per 100g	64	516	27
BN Chocolate Flavour (McVitie's)	1 biscuit (19g)	13	86	3.2
	Per 100g	71	460	17
BN Strawberry Flavour (McVitie's)	1 biscuit (19g)	15	74	1.3
	Per 100g	78	395	7
Boasters (McVitie's)	1 biscuit (19g)	11	104	6
	Per 100g	55	547	33
Bourbon Creams (Crawford's)	1 biscuit (19g)	13	94	4
	Per 100g	69	495	21
Butter Puffs (McVitie's)	1 biscuit (10g)	6	54	2.8
	Per 100g	61	523	27
Cafe Noir (McVitie's)	1 biscuit (9g)	8	39	0.6
	Per 100g	87	416	6
Chocolate Hob Nobs (McVitie's)	1 biscuit (16g)	10	81	3.9
	Per 100g	63	499	24
Chocolate Homewheat (McVitie's)	1 biscuit (17g)	11	87	4
	Per 100g	65	505	24
Custard Creams (Crawford's)	1 biscuit (11g)	1	7	0.4
	Per 100g	8	62	3

FOOD	SERVING	CARBS (g)	CALS (kcal)	FAT (g)
Digestive Creams (McVitie's)	1 biscuit (12g)	8	63	2.9
	Per 100g	68	507	23
Digestive (McVitie's)	1 biscuit (15g)	10	73	3.2
	Per 100g	68	495	22
Fig Rolls (Crawford's)	1 biscuit (15g)	11	60	1.6
	Per 100g	72	403	11
Fruit Club Biscuits (Jacob's)	1 biscuit (25g)	16	125	6
	Per 100g	62	496	25
Fruit Shortcake (McVitie's)	1 biscuit (8g)	6	39	1.8
	Per 100g	71	496	23
Garibaldi (Crawford's)	1 biscuit (10g)	7	40	1
	Per 100g	71	397	10
Ginger Nut Biscuits	1 biscuit (12g)	9	56	1.8
	Per 100g	75	455	15
Gipsy Creams (McVitie's)	1 biscuit (12g)	8	64	3.2
	Per 100g	63	515	26
Hob Nob, original (McVitie's)	1 biscuit (14g)	9	69	3.1
	Per 100g	64	484	22
Iced Gem (Jacob's)	1 biscuit (30g)	26	116	0.9
	Per 100g	86	390	3
Jaffa Cakes (McVitie's)	1 biscuit (13g)	9	48	1
	Per 100g	74	384	8
Light Digestive (McVitie's)	1 biscuit (15g)	11	70	2.4
	Per 100g	73	466	16
Lincoln Biscuits (McVitie's)	1 biscuit (8g)	6	43	2
	Per 100g	69	514	24
Marie (Crawford's)	1 biscuit (7g)	5	33	1.1
	Per 100g	76	475	16
Orange Club Biscuits (Jacob's)	1 biscuit (24g)	15	125	7
	Per 100g	62	519	28
Penguin Biscuits (McVitie's)	1 biscuit (24g)	16	131	7
	Per 100g	65	536	29
Plain Chocolate Digestive Caramels (McVitie's)	1 biscuit (17g)	11	83	3.8
	Per 100g	66	481	22

Calorie, Fat & Carbohydrate Counter

FOOD	SERVING	CARBS (g)	CALS (kcal)	FAT (g)
Plain Chocolate Ginger Nuts (McVitie's)	1 biscuit (14g)	10	70	2.9
	Per 100g	72	489	20
Plain Chocolate Hob Nobs (McVitie's)	1 biscuit (19g)	12	96	5
	Per 100g	63	498	24
Plain Chocolate Homewheat (McVitie's)	1 biscuit (17g)	12	88	4
	Per 100g	66	507	24
Real Chocolate Chip Cookies (Heinz Weight Watchers)	2 cookies (23g)	15	98	3.7
	Per 100g	66	427	16
Rich Tea Biscuits (McVitie's)	1 biscuit (8g)	6	39	1.3
	Per 100g	76	475	16
Snack Breakpack (Cadbury's)	1 biscuit (10g)	7	53	2.7
	Per 100g	64	525	27
Snack Shortcake (Cadbury's)	1 biscuit (8g)	5	42	2.2
	Per 100g	64	525	27
Stem Ginger Cookies (Heinz Weight Watchers)	1 biscuit (12g)	8	46	1.5
	Per 100g	65	399	13
Sultana & Cinnamon Cookies (Heinz Weight Watchers)	1 biscuit (12g)	8	46	1.4
	Per 100g	67	398	12

FOOD	SERVING	CARBS (g)	CALS (kcal)	FAT (g)

CAKES

Cakes – non-branded (average)

FOOD	SERVING	CARBS (g)	CALS (kcal)	FAT (g)
Angel	average slice (50g)	41	181	0.5
	Per 100g	82	362	1
Apricot crumble tea cake	average slice (50g)	22	162	8
	Per 100g	44	324	15
Apple	average slice (50g)	40	252	10
	Per 100g	80	504	20
Banana	average slice (50g)	34	214	8
	Per 100g	68	428	16
Banana madeira	average slice (50g)	29	184	7
	Per 100g	58	367	14
Banana tea loaf	average slice (50g)	28	176	6
	Per 100g	57	351	12
Battenburg	average slice (50g)	25	185	9
	Per 100g	50	370	18
Bavarian chocolate	average slice (60g)	18	200	14
	Per 100g	30	332	23
Black forest	average slice (60g)	24	200	10
	Per 100g	40	331	17
Bran loaf	average slice (70g)	42	181	1.1
	Per 100g	58	254	1.6
Cake mix, sponge, homemade	average slice (50g)	27	280	8
	Per 100g	52	560	16
Carrot cake	average slice (50g)	22	201	12
	Per 100g	44	402	23
Cheesecake	average slice (60g)	18	193	12
	Per 100g	30	320	20
Cherry cake	average slice (50g)	31	192	8
	Per 100g	62	384	16
Chinese cakes	average slice (50g)	26	207	11
	Per 100g	52	415	22

Calorie, Fat & Carbohydrate Counter

FOOD	SERVING	CARBS (g)	CALS (kcal)	FAT (g)
Chocolate	average slice (60g)	33	236	10
	Per 100g	55	391	17
Christmas	average slice (60g)	34	193	6
	Per 100g	56	116	3.6
Coconut	average slice (50g)	26	217	12
	Per 100g	51	434	24
Crispie cakes	average slice (40g)	29	186	11
	Per 100g	73	464	19
Date loaf	average slice (55g)	27	158	5
	Per 100g	49	284	9
Date and walnut loaf	average slice (60g)	32	189	6
	Per 100g	53	314	10
Éclair, chocolate, bought	average slice (70g)	23	264	18
	Per 100g	32	370	25
Flan, fruit	average slice (60g)	17	113	3.6
	Per 100g	29	187	8
Fruit cake, plain	average slice (70g)	40	230	8
	Per 100g	57	330	12
Fruit cake, retail	average slice (70g)	39	225	7
	Per 100g	55	315	10
Fruit cake, iced	average slice (70g)	44	249	8
	Per 100g	62	349	11
Fruit cake, rich	average slice (70g)	43	239	8
	Per 100g	60	335	11
Gateau	average slice (85g)	37	290	14
	Per 100g	44	348	17
Gingerbread	average slice (50g)	33	190	6
	Per 100g	66	280	12
Jam fairy	average slice (50g)	30	210	9
	Per 100g	60	420	18
Jam sponge	average slice (50g)	34	156	1.3
	Per 100g	68	312	2.5
Lamington	average slice (70g)	36	233	9
	Per 100g	47	396	15

FOOD	SERVING	CARBS (g)	CALS (kcal)	FAT (g)
Madeira	average slice (40g)	24	160	7
	Per 100g	60	400	18
Madeira iced	average slice (50g)	30	185	7
	Per 100g	60	370	14
Marble	average slice (50g)	30	375	14
	Per 100g	60	750	28
Rock	1 medium (60g)	33	221	8
	Per 100g	55	367	13
Sponge cake	average slice (60g)	33	275	16
	Per 100g	55	457	27
Sponge cake, fat free	average slice (60g)	32	175	4
	Per 100g	53	291	7
Sponge, fairy	average slice (50g)	30	172	5
	Per 100g	60	344	10
Sponge, jam filled	average slice (60g)	40	182	3
	Per 100g	66	302	5
Sponge with icing	average slice (50g)	27	244	16
	Per 100g	53	488	32
Swiss roll	average slice (35g)	24	115	2.5
	Per 100g	70	334	7
Swiss roll, chocolate	average slice (25g)	15	84	3
	Per 100g	60	336	12

Cakes – brands

FOOD	SERVING	CARBS (g)	CALS (kcal)	FAT (g)
Almond Slice (Mr Kipling) each	1 slice (30g)	18	122	4
	Per 100g	59	403	13
Angel Slice cake (Co-Op)	average slice (35g)	18	131	6
	Per 100g	4	375	17
Apple Bakes (McVitie's Go Ahead)	1 cake (35g)	26	129	3
	Per 100g	75	368	8
Apple Fruit-ins (McVitie's Go Ahead)	1 cake (16g)	12	55	0.7
	Per 100g	77	353	5
Apricot Fruit-ins (McVitie's Go Ahead)	1 cake (16g)	12	57	0.7
	Per 100g	77	353	5

Calorie, Fat & Carbohydrate Counter

FOOD	SERVING	CARBS (g)	CALS (kcal)	FAT (g)
Bakewell Tart (Marks & Spencer)	1 tart (48g)	26	230	13
	Per 100g	54	480	27
Battenburg Cake	1 slice (45g)	23	168	8
	Per 100g	50	370	18
Berry Bakes (McVitie's Go Ahead)	1 bar (35g)	26	128	0.4
	Per 100g	73	365	8
Blueberry Buster Muffin (McVitie's)	1 muffin (95g)	48	408	23
	Per 100g	50	429	24
Butter Crisp (McVitie's Go Ahead)	1 cake (6g)	5	26	0.6
	Per 100g	83	441	9
Butter Madeira Moments (McVitie's)	1 piece (30g)	15	104	5
	Per 100g	53	373	17
Caramel Creams (McVitie's Go Ahead)	1 biscuit (19g)	15	86	3
	Per 100g	77	455	14
Caramel Crisp Bar (McVitie's Go Ahead)	1 bar (33g)	24	142	4
	Per 100g	73	429	13
Caramel Shortcake (Mr Kipling)	1 cake (36g)	20	178	10
	Per 100g	58	508	29
Cherry Bakewell (Mr Kipling)	1 cake (45g)	27	186	8
	Per 100g	59	414	18
Cherry Genoa Slice Cake (McVitie's)	1 slice (28g)	16	104	4
	Per 100g	57	370	14
Choc Chip Cookie (McVitie's Go Ahead)	1 biscuit (10g)	8	45	2
	Per 100g	76	453	15
Choc Chip Mini Cake Bar (McVitie's Go Ahead)	1 bar (27g)	15	93	3
	Per 100g	55	343	12
Chocolate Caramel Crunch (McVitie's Go Ahead)	1 bar (23g)	18	102	3
	Per 100g	77	443	14
Chocolate Chip Cake Bars (Mr Kipling)	1 bar (33g)	15	148	9
	Per 100g	45	448	27
Chocolate Dream Cake Bars (McVitie's Go Ahead)	1 bar (36g)	23	141	5
	Per 100g	63	391	13

FOOD	SERVING	CARBS (g)	CALS (kcal)	FAT (g)
Chocolate Indulgence Muffin (McVitie's Go Ahead)	1 muffin (75g)	44	254	7
	Per 100g	58	338	9
Chunky Choc Chip Muffin (McVitie's)	1 muffin (94g)	47	393	20
	Per 100g	51	418	22
Coconut Madeira Moments (McVitie's)	1 piece (30g)	15	117	5
	Per 100g	52	386	18
Danish Pastries	1 pastry (110g)	57	411	20
	Per 100g	51	374	18
Dark Fruit Cake Sultana Slice (McVitie's)	1 slice (30g)	16	97	3
	Per 100g	58	347	11
Double Caramel Cake Bars (McVitie's Go Ahead)	1 slice (30g)	20	92	1.2
	Per 100g	65	302	4
Double Choc Muffin Loaf Cake (McVitie's Go Ahead)	1 slice (30g)	18	94	2
	Per 100g	60	311	7
Double Chocolate Cake Bars (McVitie's Go Ahead)	1 bar (30g)	20	92	1
	Per 100g	66	306	4
Doughnuts, jam	1 Doughnut (75g)	37	252	11
	Per 100g	49	336	15
Doughnuts, ring	1 Doughnut (60g)	28	238	13
	Per 100g	47	397	22
Flake Cakes (Cadbury's)	1 cake (26g)	14	114	6
	Per 100g	54	439	22
Fruit & Nut Crisp Bar (McVitie's Go Ahead)	1 bar (23g)	17	99	3
	Per 100g	71	431	14
Galaxy Cake Bar (McVitie's)	1 bar (30g)	18	150	8
	Per 100g	58	494	27
Galaxy Caramel Cake Bars (McVitie's)	1 bar (33g)	20	147	7
	Per 100g	59	444	21
Ginger Crisp (McVitie's Go Ahead)	1 biscuit (6g)	5	26	0.5
	Per 100g	83	438	9
Golden Crunch (McVitie's Go Ahead)	1 biscuit (8g)	6	34	0.8
	Per 100g	75	419	10

Calorie, Fat & Carbohydrate Counter

FOOD	SERVING	CARBS (g)	CALS (kcal)	FAT (g)
Homebake Chocolate Cake (McVitie's)	1 slice (50g)	28	178	7
	Per 100g	55	355	14
Homebake Genoa Cake (McVitie's)	1 slice (50g)	28	192	8
	Per 100g	56	383	16
Homebake Lemon Cake (McVitie's)	1 slice (50g)	27	192	9
	Per 100g	54	384	18
Homebake Marble Cake (McVitie's)	1 slice (50g)	29	220	10
	Per 100g	57	441	19
Jaffa Cakes Muffin (McVitie's)	1 muffin (101g)	58	415	19
	Per 100g	57	411	19
Jam Tarts	1 slice (90g)	56	342	14
	Per 100g	62	380	15
Jamaica Ginger Bar Cake (McVitie's)	1 mini cake (33g)	20	128	5
	Per 100g	60	388	15
Kensington Slab Cake (McVitie's)	1 slice (50g)	29	188	7
	Per 100g	57	375	14
Lemon Curd Mini Cake Bar (McVitie's)	1 cake (33g)	20	129	5
	Per 100g	61	390	14
Lemon Madeira Moments (McVitie's)	1 slice (50g)	28	189	8
	Per 100g	55	378	15
Lemon Slices (Mr Kipling) each	1 slice (90g)	52	375	14
	Per 100g	58	417	16
M&M's Chocolate Brownie (McVitie's)	1 brownie (89g)	52	408	20
	Per 100g	59	458	23
Madeira Cake	1 slice (40g)	24	157	7
	Per 100g	59	393	17
Milky Way Cake Bar (McVitie's)	1 bar (26g)	14	138	9
	Per 100g	54	530	33
Mince Pies (Mr Kipling)	1 pie (62g)	35	231	9
	Per 100g	54	372	14
Raspin Jack (McVitie's)	1 portion (30g)	18	145	7
	Per 100g	60	477	24

FOOD	SERVING	CARBS (g)	CALS (kcal)	FAT (g)
Strawberry Dream Cake Bar (McVitie's Go Ahead)	1 cake (33g)	22	104	2
	Per 100g	65	314	6
Strawberry Mallow (McVitie's Go Ahead)	1 biscuit (18g)	13	69	2
	Per 100g	71	385	10
Strawberry Milky Way Cake Bar (McVitie's)	1 bar (28g)	15	146	9
	Per 100g	53	520	32
Syrup Jack (McVitie's)	1 portion (30g)	18	146	8
	Per 100g	59	483	25
Toffee Bar Cake (McVitie's)	1 slice (85g)	52	295	8
	Per 100g	61	382	14
Toffee Temptation Muffin (McVitie's Go Ahead)	1 muffin (70g)	42	256	9
	Per 100g	60	347	10

FOOD	SERVING	CARBS (g)	CALS (kcal)	FAT (g)

CHOCOLATES AND SWEETS

Confectionery – non-branded (average)

FOOD	SERVING	CARBS (g)	CALS (kcal)	FAT (g)
Almonds, chocolate-coated	7 (about 30g)	11	159	12
	Per 100g	39	561	43
Almonds, sugar-coated	8 (30g)	20	128	5
	Per 100g	69	451	18
Butterscotch	4 pieces (30g)	27	111	1
	Per 100g	93	392	3.5
Candy corn	20 pieces (about 30g)	25	102	0.6
	Per 100g	89	360	2.1
Caramel, plain or chocolate	30g	22	112	2.9
	Per 100g	76	395	10
Chocolate, milk	30g	16	146	9
	Per 100g	56	515	32
Chocolate, semisweet	30g	16	142	10
	Per 100g	56	501	35
Coconut, chocolate-coated	30g	20	123	5
	Per 100g	71	434	17
Fudge, chocolate	30g	21	112	3.4
	Per 100g	74	395	12
Fudge, chocolate, chocolate-coated	30g	21	120	5
	Per 100g	72	423	16
Fudge, vanilla	30g	21	111	3.1
	Per 100g	74	392	11
Ginger root, crystallised, candied	30g	24	95	0.1
	Per 100g	86	335	0.4
Gumdrops	30g	25	100	tr
	Per 100g	88	353	tr
Hard candy	30g	27	108	0.3
	Per 100g	96	381	1.1
Jelly beans	10 (30g)	26	103	0.1
	Per 100g	92	363	0.4

FOOD	SERVING	CARBS (g)	CALS (kcal)	FAT (g)
Mints, chocolate-coated	12 mini (about 30g)	23	115	2.9
	Per 100g	80	406	10
Mints, plain	30g	25	102	0.6
	Per 100g	89	360	2.1
Nougat and caramel candy bar	30g	20	116	3.9
	Per 100g	72	409	14
Peanut bars	30g	13	144	9
	Per 100g	47	508	32
Peanut brittle	30g	23	118	2.9
	Per 100g	80	416	10
Peanuts, chocolate-coated	12 (about 30g)	11	157	12
	Per 100g	39	554	41
Raisins, chocolate-coated	30 (about 30g)	20	119	5
	Per 100g	69	420	17
Vanilla creams, chocolate-coated	30g	20	122	5
	Per 100g	69	430	17

Confectionery – brands

FOOD	SERVING	CARBS (g)	CALS (kcal)	FAT (g)
Aero Creamy White (Nestlé)	1 bar (48g)	27	254	14
	Per 100g	57	530	30
Aero Mint (Nestlé)	1 bar (46g)	28	254	13
	Per 100g	60	552	29
After Eight Mints (Nestlé)	1 mint (8g)	6	34	1
	Per 100g	72	419	13
Allora (Cadbury's)	1 bar (28g)	14	151	10
	Per 100g	51	540	34
Boost (Cadbury's)	1 bar (55g)	34	297	16
	Per 100g	62	540	29
Bounty (Mars)	1 bar (58g)	32	275	15
	Per 100g	56	474	26
Bourneville Chocolate (Cadbury's)	1 bar (45g)	27	223	12
	Per 100g	60	495	27
California Dreaming (Cadbury's)	1 bar (52g)	31	250	12
	Per 100g	60	480	24

Calorie, Fat & Carbohydrate Counter

FOOD	SERVING	CARBS (g)	CALS (kcal)	FAT (g)
Caramel (Cadbury's)	1 bar (50g)	31	240	12
	Per 100g	61	480	24
Chocolate Buttons (Cadbury's)	1 pack (65g)	37	341	19
	Per 100g	57	525	29
Chocolate Cream (Cadbury's)	1 bar (51g)	35	217	8
	Per 100g	69	425	15
Chocolate M & Ms (Mars)	1 pack (45g)	32	216	9
	Per 100g	70	481	21
Chomp (Cadbury's)	1 bar (27g)	18	126	5
	Per 100g	68	465	20
Crunchie (Cadbury's)	1 bar (41g)	30	193	7
	Per 100g	72	470	18
Curly Wurly (Cadbury's)	1 bar (29g)	20	131	5
	Per 100g	70	450	17
Dairy Box Assortment (Nestlé)	1 box (125g)	76	589	28
	Per 100g	61	471	22
Dairy Milk Chocolate (Cadbury's)	1 bar (49g)	28	260	15
	Per 100g	57	530	30
Dairy Milk Tasters (Cadbury's)	1 pack (49g)	28	255	14
	Per 100g	57	520	29
Dairy Milk Orange (Cadbury's)	1 bar (50g)	28	257	15
	Per 100g	56	514	30
Double Decker (Cadbury's)	1 bar (65g)	42	302	14
	Per 100g	65	465	21
Double Fudge Dream (Cadbury's)	1 bar (28g)	17	139	7
	Per 100g	61	495	25
Drifter (Nestlé)	1 bar (61g)	40	296	13
	Per 100g	66	486	22
Flake (Cadbury's)	1 bar (34g)	19	180	11
	Per 100g	56	530	31
Freddo (Cadbury's)	1 bar (17g)	10	89	5
	Per 100g	57	525	29
Fruit & Nut Chocolate (Cadbury's)	1 bar (49g)	27	238	13
	Per 100g	55	485	26

FOOD	SERVING	CARBS (g)	CALS (kcal)	FAT (g)
Fruit & Nut Tasters (Cadbury's)	1 pack (46g)	26	232	13
	Per 100g	57	505	29
Fruit Pastilles (Rowntree)	12 sweets (53g)	44	184	0
	Per 100g	83	348	0
Fudge (Cadbury's)	1 bar (26g)	19	116	4
	Per 100g	72	445	16
Fuse (Cadbury's)	1 bar (49g)	28	238	12
	Per 100g	58	485	25
Galaxy Caramel (Mars)	1 bar (48g)	29	233	12
	Per 100g	60	485	25
Galaxy Fruit & Nut (Mars)	1 bar (47g)	27	235	13
	Per 100g	58	501	28
Galaxy Hazelnut (Mars)	1 bar (47g)	22	267	18
	Per 100g	46	569	39
Galaxy Milk Chocolate (Mars)	1 bar (75g)	45	405	24
	Per 100g	60	540	32
Heroes (Cadbury's)	1 box (125g)	76	631	33
	Per 100g	61	505	26
Jellytots (Nestlé)	1 bar (42g)	37	145	0
	Per 100g	87	346	0
Kit Kat (Nestlé)	1 bar (49g)	29	246	13
	Per 100g	60	502	26
Lion Bar (Nestlé)	1 bar (56g)	37	270	12
	Per 100g	66	482	22
Maltesers (Mars)	1 bar (41g)	25	199	9
	Per 100g	61	486	23
Marble (Cadbury's)	1 bar (46g)	25	246	14
	Per 100g	55	535	31
Mars Bar (Mars)	1 bar (59g)	41	281	11
	Per 100g	70	477	18
Milk Chocolate Aero (Nestlé)	1 bar (39g)	22	202	11
	Per 100g	57	518	29
Milk Chocolate Yorkie (Nestlé)	1 bar (70g)	41	368	21
	Per 100g	59	526	30

Calorie, Fat & Carbohydrate Counter

FOOD	SERVING	CARBS (g)	CALS (kcal)	FAT (g)
Milk Tray (Cadbury's)	1 box (125g)	76	625	33
	Per 100g	61	500	26
Milky Way (Mars)	1 bar (26g)	19	116	4
	Per 100g	72	447	16
Mint Chocolate Aero (Nestlé)	1 bar (48g)	27	252	14
	Per 100g	57	526	29
Munchies (Nestlé)	1 pack (51g)	32	254	13
	Per 100g	63	498	26
Nobble (Cadbury's)	1 bar (30g)	21	138	5
	Per 100g	69	460	18
Nuts about Caramel (Cadbury's)	1 bar (56g)	32	277	15
	Per 100g	58	495	27
Old Jamaica (Cadbury's)	1 bar (101g)	58	465	23
	Per 100g	57	460	23
Orange Cream (Cadbury's)	1 bar (60g)	41	255	9
	Per 100g	69	425	15
Peppermint Cream (Cadbury's)	1 bar (51g)	35	217	8
	Per 100g	69	425	15
Picnic (Cadbury's)	1 bar (48g)	28	228	12
	Per 100g	59	475	24
Quality Street (Nestlé)	1 box (125g)	84	583	26
	Per 100g	67	466	21
Revels (Mars)	1 pack (35g)	23	171	8
	Per 100g	66	489	23
Roses (Cadbury's)	1 box (125g)	76	619	31
	Per 100g	61	495	25
Snickers (Mars)	1 bar (64g)	35	321	18
	Per 100g	55	502	28
Toffee Crisp (Nestlé)	1 bar (49g)	30	242	13
	Per 100g	62	494	26
Topic (Mars)	1 bar (48g)	27	236	12
	Per 100g	57	492	26
Time Out (Cadbury's)	1 finger (18g)	5	97	11
	Per 100g	29	540	62

FOOD	SERVING	CARBS (g)	CALS (kcal)	FAT (g)
Twirl (Cadbury's)	1 bar (44g)	25	231	13
	Per 100g	56	525	30
Twix (Mars)	1 finger (29g)	19	144	7
	Per 100g	64	495	24
Walnut Whip (Nestlé)	1 pack (34g)	18	165	9
	Per 100g	52	486	25
White Chocolate Buttons (Nestlé)	1 pack (33g)	19	179	10
	Per 100g	58	542	31
Wholenut Chocolate (Cadbury's)	1 bar (50g)	25	270	17
	Per 100g	49	540	34
Wholenut Tasters (Cadbury's)	1 pack (45g)	20	250	17
	Per 100g	44	555	38
Wispa (Cadbury's)	1 bar (39g)	21	215	13
	Per 100g	54	550	34
Wispa Gold (Cadbury's)	1 bar (51g)	29	263	15
	Per 100g	56	515	30
Wispa Mint (Cadbury's)	1 bar (50g)	30	275	17
	Per 100g	60	550	34
Yowie (Cadbury's)	1 bar (70g)	40	368	20
	Per 100g	57	525	29

FOOD	SERVING	CARBS (g)	CALS (kcal)	FAT (g)

DESSERTS

Desserts – non-branded (average)

FOOD	SERVING	CARBS (g)	CALS (kcal)	FAT (g)
Apple pie	1 slice (about 115g)	45	302	13
	Per 100g	39	263	11
Banana cream pie, homemade	1 slice (about 115g)	40	285	12
	Per 100g	35	248	10
Blackberry pie	1 slice (about 115g)	41	287	13
	Per 100g	36	250	11
Blueberry pie	1 slice (about 115g)	41	286	13
	Per 100g	36	249	11
Bread & butter pudding	1 slice (about 115g)	21	184	9
	Per 100g	18	160	8
Chocolate cream pie	1 slice (about 115g)	30	264	15
	Per 100g	26	230	13
Christmas pudding	1 slice (about 115g)	58	335	12
	Per 100g	50	291	10
Cream horns	1 oz (28g)	7	122	10
	Per 100g	26	435	36
Creme Caramel	1 serving (about 115g)	24	125	2
	Per 100g	21	109	2
Custard tarts	1 tart (94g)	31	260	14
	Per 100g	33	277	15
Fruit trifle	1 trifle (50g)	10	83	5
	Per 100g	19	166	9
Lemon meringue pie	1 slice (about 115g)	40	268	11
	Per 100g	35	233	10
Mince pie	1 pie (about 50g)	28	183	8
	Per 100g	56	366	15
Peach pie	1 slice (about 115g)	45	301	13
	Per 100g	39	262	11
Pecan pie	1 slice (about 115g)	53	431	24
	Per 100g	46	375	21

FOOD	SERVING	CARBS (g)	CALS (kcal)	FAT (g)
Pumpkin pie	1 slice (about 115g)	28	241	13
	Per 100g	24	210	11
Raisin pie	1 slice (about 115g)	51	319	13
	Per 100g	44	277	11
Rhubarb pie	1 slice (about 115g)	45	299	13
	Per 100g	39	260	11
Strawberry pie	1 slice (about 115g)	29	184	7
	Per 100g	25	160	6
Sweet potato pie	1 slice (about 115g)	27	243	13
	Per 100g	23	211	11

Puddings – brands

FOOD	SERVING	CARBS (g)	CALS (kcal)	FAT (g)
Apple Crumble with Sultanas (Heinz Weight Watchers)	1 dessert (110g)	38	196	4
	Per 100g	34	178	4
Apple Turnovers (Co-Op)	1 Turnover (77g)	27	308	21
	Per 100g	35	400	27
Apple & Blackberry Pie (Somerfield)	1/4 pie (106g)	38	280	13
	Per 100g	50	330	13
Banana Flavoured Custard Dessert (Ambrosia)	1 pack (135g)	22	136	4
	Per 100g	16	101	3
Banoffee Pie (Tesco)	1 pie (112g)	51	381	18
	Per 100g	46	340	16
Bramley Apple Pies, deep filled (Mr Kipling)	1 pie (66g)	34	220	9
	Per 100g	51	333	13
Bramley Apple & Custard Lattice Topped Pies (Mr Kipling)	1 pie (64g)	31	217	9
	Per 100g	48	339	15
Carrot Cake (Pret á Manger)	1 cake 110g	53	419	21
	Per 100g	48	381	19
Chocolate Cheesecake (Heinz Weight Watchers)	1 cheesecake (p5g)	20	143	4
	Per 100g	21	151	4
Chocolate Cheesecake (Marks & Spencer)	1 oz (28g)	11	106	6
	Per 100g	40	380	22

Calorie, Fat & Carbohydrate Counter

FOOD	SERVING	CARBS (g)	CALS (kcal)	FAT (g)
Chocolate Chip Cheesecake (Marks & Spencer)	1 oz (28g)	11	109	7
	Per 100g	40	391	24
Chocolate Eclairs fresh cream (Co-op)	1 éclair (8g)	6	38	2
	Per 100g	71	470	19
Chocolate Mousse (Heinz Weight Watchers)	1 pot (54g)	6	52	2
	Per 100g	10	97	4
Chocolate Mousse (Somerfield)	1 pot (60g)	24	309	22
	Per 100g	40	515	36
Chocolate Truffle cake (Somerfield)	1 oz (28g)	14	136	8
	Per 100g	51	845	28
Creamed Macaroni Pudding (Ambrosia)	1 can (425g)	62	374	7
	Per 100g	15	88	2
Creamed Macaroni Pudding (Co-Op)	1 can (425g)	68	383	9
	Per 100g	16	90	2
Creamed Rice Pudding (Ambrosia)	1 can (425g)	65	383	8
	Per 100g	15	90	2
Creamed Rice Pudding (Co-Op)	1 can (170g)	27	153	3
	Per 100g	16	90	2
Creamed Sago Pudding (Ambrosia)	1 can (425g)	58	336	7
	Per 100g	13	79	2
Creamed Sago Pudding (Co-Op)	1 can (425g)	68	361	9
	Per 100g	16	85	2
Creamy Rice (Shape)	1 serving (175g)	27	149	2
	Per 100g	16	85	1
Creamy Rice with Strawberry Crunch Dessert (Ambrosia)	1 pack (205g)	47	297	9
	Per 100g	23	145	4
Creamy Rice with Tropical Crunch Dessert (Ambrosia)	1 pack (210g)	49	307	9
	Per 100g	24	146	4
Creme Caramel (Organic Evernat)	1 oz (28g)	6	37	1
	Per 100g	21	132	4

FOOD	SERVING	CARBS (g)	CALS (kcal)	FAT (g)
Forest Fruits Crispy Fruit Slice, Go Ahead, (McVitie's)	1 biscuit (14g)	10	56	1
	Per 100g	73	400	9
Forest Fruits Flavour Hot 'n' Fruity Custard Pot (Bird's)	1 pot (174g)	32	171	4
	Per 100g	19	98	3
Fruit Cocktail Luxury Devonshire Trifle (St Ivel)	1 trifle (125g)	28	211	10
	Per 100g	23	169	8
Fruit Cocktail Trifle (Shape)	1 trifle (115g)	23	136	3
	Per 100g	20	118	3
Fruit Cocktail Trifle (St Ivel)	1 pot (140g)	27	113	0.3
	Per 100g	19	81	0.2
Ginger Sponge Pudding with Plum Sauce (Waitrose)	1 pudding (120g)	62	424	18
	Per 100g	52	353	15
Golden Syrup sponge pudding (Co-Op)	1 can (300g)	141	945	39
	Per 100g	47	315	13
Gooseberry Crumble (Marks & Spencer)	1 serving (133g)	56	379	14
	Per 100g	43	285	11
Gooseberry Pie, Puff pastry (Marks & Spencer)	1 pie (135g)	42	311	15
	Per 100g	32	230	11
Iced Dessert, Chocolate & Honeycomb Pieces, (Heinz Weight Watchers)	1 pot (57g)	15	92	3
	Per 100g	26	159	4
Iced Dessert, Raspberry Swirl (Heinz Weight Watchers)	1 scoop (60g)	14	74	2
	Per 100g	24	124	3
Iced Dessert, Toffee Flavour Fudge Swirl (Heinz Weight Watchers)	1 pot (57g)	13	82	3
	Per 100g	23	143	5
Iced Dessert, Toffee Flavour & Toffee Sauce (Heinz Weight Watchers)	1 pot (57g)	15	93	3
	Per 100g	26	163	5

Calorie, Fat & Carbohydrate Counter

FOOD	SERVING	CARBS (g)	CALS (kcal)	FAT (g)
Iced Dessert, Vanilla Flavour (Heinz Weight Watchers)	1 scoop (60g)	12	74	2
	Per 100g	20	124	4
Iced Dessert, Vanilla & Raspberry Compote (Heinz Weight Watchers)	1 scoop (60g)	15	88	3
	Per 100g	23	142	4
Iced Dessert, Vanilla & Strawberry Compote (Heinz Weight Watchers)	1 pot (57g)	13	81	2
	Per 100g	24	142	4
Iced Topped Mince Pies, (Marks & Spencer)	1 pie (47g)	31	181	6
	Per 100g	66	385	13
Instant Desert Powder, made with skimmed milk	1 oz (28g)	4	27	0.9
	Per 100g	15	97	3
Instant Desert Powder, made with whole milk	1 oz (28g)	4	35	2
	Per 100g	15	125	6
Lemon Curd Sponge Pudding (Heinz)	1/4 can (78g)	37	236	9
	Per 100g	47	302	12
Lemon Curd Tarts (Asda)	1 tart (35g)	23	139	4
	Per 100g	66	396	12
Lemon Meringue Iced Desert (Marks & Spencer)	1 oz (28g)	10	47	0.7
	Per 100g	34	167	3
Lemon Meringue Pies, (Mr Kipling)	1 cake (51g)	31	184	6
	Per 100g	60	360	12
Lemon Mousse Desert (Sainsbury's)	1 oz (28g)	6	51	3
	Per 100g	21	182	10
Lemon Pancakes (Marks & Spencer)	1 oz (28g)	12	85	4
	Per 100g	41	305	14
Lemon Puddings (Sainsbury's)	1 pudding (110g)	46	304	12
	Per 100g	42	276	11
Low Fat Rice Pudding (Ambrosia)	1 pot (150g)	24	129	1
	Per 100g	16	86	0.9
Luxury Mince Pies (Marks & Spencer)	1 pie (59g)	35	227	9
	Per 100g	59	385	15

FOOD	SERVING	CARBS (g)	CALS (kcal)	FAT (g)
Mandarin Fruit Luxuries, (Co-Op)	1 tart (33g)	10	81	4
	Per 100g	29	245	13
Mandarin dessert, (Marks & Spencer)	1 oz (28g)	6	35	1
	Per 100g	20	125	5
Milk Chocolate Flavoured Custard Dessert (Ambrosia)	1 pack (135g)	30	169	4
	Per 100g	22	125	3
Mince Pies, puff pastry, (Marks & Spencer)	1 pie (47g)	26	190	9
	Per 100g	56	405	19
Mince Pies (Mr Kipling)	1 pie (62g)	35	231	9
	Per 100g	60	372	15
Natural rice dessert, (Shape)	1 pot (175g)	27	149	2
	Per 100g	16	85	1
Pancakes, Scotch	1 pancake (50g)	22	146	6
	Per 100g	44	292	12
Passion fruit & orange gateau, (Marks & Spencer)	1 serving (103g)	27	221	12
	Per 100g	26	215	12
Raspberry Luxury Devonshire Trifle (St Ivel)	1 trifle (125g)	27	208	10
	Per 100g	22	166	8
Raspberry Trifle (St Ivel)	1 trifle (113g)	24	195	10
	Per 100g	21	173	9
Rhubarb and Custard Pies (Asda)	1 pie (56g)	31	181	6
	Per 100g	55	324	10
Rhubarb Crumble (Co-Op)	1 crumble (440g)	185	1078	31
	Per 100g	42	245	7
Rice Pudding, No Added Sugar, Low Fat (Heinz Weight Watchers)	1 can (424g)	48	310	6
	Per 100g	11	73	2
Rich Chocolate Pudding (Tryton Foods)	1 serving (110g)	46	300	11
	Per 100g	42	273	10
Sherry Trifle (Co-Op)	1/4 trifle (188g)	45	320	13
	Per 100g	24	170	8

Calorie, Fat & Carbohydrate Counter

FOOD	SERVING	CARBS (g)	CALS (kcal)	FAT (g)
Sponge Pudding, Banoffee Canned (Heinz)	1/4 can (78g)	36	239	10
	Per 100g	47	307	12
Sponge Pudding, Lemon Curd Canned (Heinz)	1/4 can (78g)	37	236	9
	Per 100g	47	302	12
Sponge Pudding, Spotted Dick Canned (Heinz)	1/4 can (78g)	37	244	10
	Per 100g	50	325	13
Sponge Pudding, Sticky Toffee Canned (Heinz)	1/4 can (78g)	35	235	10
	Per 100g	45	305	13
Sponge Pudding, Strawberry Jam Canned (Heinz)	1/4 can (80g)	41	230	6
	Per 100g	51	281	8
Sponge Pudding, Treacle Canned (Heinz)	1/4 can (80g)	39	222	6
	Per 100g	49	277	8
Sticky Toffee Pudding (Co-Op)	1/4 pudding (90g)	36	320	18
	Per 100g	40	355	20
Strawberry Cheesecake (Heinz Weight Watchers)	1 cheesecake (90g)	23	148	3.6
	Per 100g	26	164	4
Strawberry Flavour Custard Desert, (Ambrosia)	1 pack (135g)	22	136	4
	Per 100g	16	101	3
Strawberry Flavour Hot 'n' Fruity Custard Pot (Bird's)	1 oz (28g)	5	28	0.7
	Per 100g	19	99	3
Strawberry Luxury Devonshire Trifle (St Ivel)	1 trifle (125g)	27	208	10
	Per 100g	22	166	8
Strawberry Trifle (Shape St Ivel)	1 pot (115g)	23	137	3
	Per 100g	20	119	3
Strawberry Trifle (St Ivel)	1 trifle (113g)	24	114	10
	Per 100g	21	172	9
Summer Pudding (Waitrose)	1 pot (120g)	30	125	0.5
	Per 100g	23	105	0.4
Syrup Puddings (Co-Op)	1 pudding (170g)	65	604	36
	Per 100g	38	355	21
Tarte Au Choc Noir Blanc (Marks & Spencer)	1 oz (28g)	11	151	11
	Per 100g	40	540	40

FOOD	SERVING	CARBS (g)	CALS (kcal)	FAT (g)
Tarte Citron (Marks & Spencer)	1 oz (28g)	10	98	6
	Per 100g	36	350	21
Tarte aux pommes (Marks & Spencer)	1 oz (28g)	11	81	4
	Per 100g	40	290	14
Toffee Chocolate Dessert (Heinz Weight Watchers)	1 desert (92g)	31	169	3
	Per 100g	33	184	4
Toffee Flavoured Custard Dessert (Ambrosia)	1 pack (135g)	22	139	4
	Per 100g	17	103	3
Traditional Rice Pudding with Sultanas & Nutmeg (Ambrosia)	1 pack (425g)	71	446	12
	Per 100g	17	105	3
Treacle Tart (Co-Op)	1 tart (41g)	29	162	4.5
	Per 100g	70	395	11
White Chocolate Flavoured Custard Dessert (Ambrosia)	1 pack (135g)	26	150	4
	Per 100g	19	111	3

7
Fast food

Calorie, Fat & Carbohydrate Counter

FOOD	SERVING	CARBS (g)	CALS (kcal)	FAT (g)
BURGER KING				
Apple pie	1 serving	44	311	14
Bacon bits	1 pkt	0	16	1
Bagels				
Plain	1 bagel	44	272	6
W/cream cheese	1 bagel	45	370	16
Barbecue sauce	28g	9	36	0
Biscuit, plain	1 serving	42	332	17
Breakfast				
French toast sticks	1 serving	60	440	27
Scrambled egg platter, regular	1 serving	44	549	34
Scrambled egg platter, w/bacon	1 serving	44	610	39
Scrambled egg platter, w/sausage	1 serving	47	768	53
Breakfast sandwich				
Bagel, w/bacon, egg and cheese	1 serving	46	453	20
Bagel, w/egg and cheese	1 serving	46	407	16
Bagel, w/ham, egg and cheese	1 serving	46	438	17
Bagel, w/sausage, egg, and cheese	1 serving	49	626	36
Biscuit, w/bacon	1 serving	42	378	20
Biscuit, w/bacon and egg	1 serving	43	467	27
Biscuit, w/sausage	1 serving	44	478	29
Biscuit, w/sausage and egg	1 serving	45	568	36
Croissan'wich' w/bacon, egg, and cheese	1 serving	19	353	23
Croissan'wich' w/egg and cheese	1 serving	19	315	20
Croissan'wich' w/ham, egg and cheese	1 serving	20	351	22
Croissan'wich' w/sausage, egg and cheese	1 serving	22	534	40
Cheeseburger				
Bacon, double	1 serving	26	515	31
Bacon, double, 'Deluxe'	1 serving	28	592	39

FOOD	SERVING	CARBS (g)	CALS (kcal)	FAT (g)
Barbecue bacon, double	1 serving	31	536	31
Deluxe	1 serving	29	390	23
Double	1 serving	29	483	27
Mushroom Swiss double	1 serving	27	473	27
Regular	1 serving	28	318	15
Whopper double w/cheese	1 serving	47	935	61
Whopper w/cheese	1 serving	47	706	44
Chicken Sandwich regular	1 serving	56	685	40
Cream Cheese	28g	1	98	10
Croissant	1 serving	18	180	10
Croutons	7g	5	31	1

Danish

Apple cinnamon	1 serving	62	390	13
Cheese	1 serving	60	406	16
Cinnamon raisin	1 serving	63	449	18

Fish sandwich

Fillet, 'Ocean Catch'	1 serving	49	495	25
French Fries, medium order	1 serving	43	372	20

Hamburger

Deluxe	1 serving	28	344	19
Regular	1 serving	28	272	11
Whopper	1 serving	45	614	36
Whopper double	1 serving	45	844	53
Honey Sauce	28g	23	91	0
Lettuce	21g	0	3	0
Mayonnaise	28g	2	194	21

Calorie, Fat & Carbohydrate Counter

FOOD	SERVING	CARBS (g)	CALS (kcal)	FAT (g)
Milkshake				
Chocolate	1 serving	49	326	10
Chocolate, syrup added	1 serving	68	409	11
Strawberry, syrup added	1 serving	66	394	10
Vanilla	1 serving	51	334	10
Muffin				
Blueberry, mini	1 serving	37	292	14
Lemon poppyseed, mini	1 serving	33	318	18
Mustard	1 serving	0	2	0
Onion	7g	1	5	0
Onion rings	1 serving	38	339	19
Pickle	14g	0	1	0
Potatoes, Hash Brown	1 serving	25	213	12
Ranch Sauce	28g	2	171	18
Salad				
Chef's w/o dressing	1 serving	7	178	9
Chunky chicken, w/o dressing	1 serving	8	142	4
Garden, w/o dressing	1 serving	8	95	5
Side salad, w/o dressing	1 serving	5	25	0
Salad dressing				
Blue cheese (Newman's Own)	1 pkt	2	300	32
French (Newman's Own)	1 pkt	23	290	22
Italian, reduced calorie (Newman's Own)	1 pkt	3	170	18
Olive oil and vinegar (Newman's Own)	1 pkt	2	310	33
Ranch (Newman's Own)	1 pkt	4	350	37
Thousand Island (Newman's Own)	1 pkt	15	290	26
Sweet and sour sauce	28g	11	45	0
Tartar sauce	28g	2	134	14
Tomato	28g	1	6	0

FOOD	SERVING	CARBS (g)	CALS (kcal)	FAT (g)
KENTUCKY FRIED CHICKEN				
Chicken				
Breast, centre, 'Extra Tasty Crispy'	1 serving (136g)	12	342	20
	Per 100g	9	251	15
Breast, centre, 'Hot & Spicy'	1 serving (120g)	16	382	25
	Per 100g	13	318	21
Breast, centre, 'Original Recipe'	1 serving (100g)	8	260	14
	Per 100g	8	260	14
Breast, side, 'Extra Tasty Crispy'	1 serving (106g)	14	343	22
	Per 100g	13	324	21
Breast, side, 'Hot & Spicy'	1 serving (116g)	18	398	27
	Per 100g	16	343	23
Breast, side, 'Skinfree Crispy'	1 serving (120g)	11	293	17
	Per 100g	9	244	14
Colonel's' Choice Fillet Tower Burger	1 serving (285g)	57	661	31
	Per 100g	20	232	11
Colonel's' Choice Fillets Sandwich	1 serving (215g)	41	473	19
	Per 100g	19	220	9
Crispy strips	1 serving (110g)	17	295	17
	Per 100g	15	268	15
Dark meat quarter, w/o skin, 'Rotisserie Gold'	1 serving (116g)	0	217	12
	Per 100g	0	187	10
Dark meat quarter, w/skin, 'Rotisserie Gold'	1 serving (145g)	1	333	24
	Per 100g	0.7	230	17
Drumstick, Hot & Spicy'	1 serving (64g)	10	190	11
	Per 100g	16	297	17
Drumstick, Original Recipe'	1 serving (48g)	4	125	7
	Per 100g	9	260	15
Drumstick, 'Extra Tasty Crispy'	1 serving (64g)	8	190	11
	Per 100g	13	297	17
Hot wings (3)	1 serving (130g)	51	394	27
	Per 100g	39	303	21

Calorie, Fat & Carbohydrate Counter

FOOD	SERVING	CARBS (g)	CALS (kcal)	FAT (g)
Hot Wings (6)	1 serving (134g)	18	471	33
	Per 100g	13	351	25
keel, 'Original Recipe'	1 serving (100g)	5	346	12
	Per 100g	5	346	12
Kentucky Nuggets'	1 nugget (16g)	2.2	46	2.9
	Per 100g	14	288	18
Popcorn Chicken	1 serving (145g)	19	384	23
	Per 100g	13	265	16
Rib, 'Original Recipe'	1 serving (100g)	9	264	6
	Per 100g	9	264	6
Spicy Chicken Bites' small	1 serving (120g)	5	248	12
	Per 100g	4	207	10
Thigh, 'Extra Tasty Crispy'	1 serving (117g)	7	370	25
	Per 100g	6	316	21
Thigh, 'Hot & Spicy'	1 serving (106g)	13	370	27
	Per 100g	12	349	25
Thigh, 'Original Recipe'	1 serving (90g)	5	251	18
	Per 100g	6	279	20
Thigh, 'Skinfree Crispy'	1 serving	9	256	17
	Per 100g			
Twister	1 serving (225g)	43	524	29
	Per 100g	19	233	13
Wing, 'Extra Tasty Crispy'	1 serving (53g)	10	200	13
	Per 100g	19	377	25
Wing, 'Hot & Spicy'	1 serving (53g)	9	210	15
	Per 100g	17	396	28
Wing, 'Original Recipe'	1 serving (53g)	4	148	10
	Per 100g	7	280	18
Zinger Sandwich	1 serving (185g)	41	446	20
	Per 100g	22	241	11
Zinger Tower Burger	1 serving (256g)	51	620	31
	Per 100g	20	242	12

FOOD	SERVING	CARBS (g)	CALS (kcal)	FAT (g)
Vegetarian				
Vegie Twister	1 serving (240g)	55	593	36
	Per 100g	23	247	15
Vegie Strips	1 serving (130g)	30	322	18
	Per 100g	23	248	14
Side orders				
BBQ beans (regular)	1 serving (110g)	20	101	0.4
	Per 100g	18	92	0.4
BBQ beans (large)	1 serving (260g)	113	569	2.3
	Per 100g	44	219	0.9
Cobette with butter	Per portion	15	101	3.5
	Per 100g	23	150	5
Cobette without butter	Per portion	15	80	1.5
	Per 100g	23	123	2.3
Coleslaw (regular)	1 serving (100g)	5	147	13
	Per 100g	5	147	13
Coleslaw (large)	1 serving (200g)	10	294	26
	Per 100g	5	147	13
Corn, on the cob	1 serving (150g)	27	222	12
	Per 100g	18	148	8
Cornbread	1 serving (60g)	25	228	13
	Per 100g	42	380	22
French Fries (regular)	Regular	36	294	15
	Per 100g	32	257	13
French Fries (large)	Large	47	382	19
	Per 100g	32	257	13
Green beans	1 serving (100g)	5	36	1
	Per 100g	5	36	1
Macaroni and cheese	1 serving (116g)	15	162	8
	Per 100g	13	140	7
Potato wedges	1 serving (92g)	25	192	9
	Per 100g	27	209	10

Calorie, Fat & Carbohydrate Counter

FOOD	SERVING	CARBS (g)	CALS (kcal)	FAT (g)
Red Beans and Rice	1 serving (109g)	114	114	3
	Per 100g	105	105	2.8
Rice, garden	1 serving (106g)	75	75	1
	Per 100g	71	71	0.9
Roll	1 serving (50g)	128	128	2
	Per 100g	256	256	4

Salad

Garden	1 serving (87g)	16	16	0
	Per 100g	18	18	0
Macaroni	1 serving (106g)	20	240	17
	Per 100g	19	226	16
Pasta	1 serving (106g)	12	130	8
	Per 100g	11	123	7
Potato	1 serving (123g)	20	175	11
	Per 100g	16	142	9
Vegetable medley	1 serving (112g)	18	120	5
	Per 100g	16	109	5

Salad dressing

Italian	1 serving (30g)	15	15	1
	Per 100g	50	50	3.3
Ranch	1 serving (30g)	170	170	18
	Per 100g	567	567	60

Dips

Barbecue Sauce	1 serving (30g)	7	35	0.6
	Per 100g	23	117	2
Honey BBQ Dip	1 serving (30g)	8	35	0
	Per 100g	28	116	0
Sour Cream & Chive Dip	1 serving (30g)	0.9	98	11
	Per 100g	2.9	328	35
Sweet and sour dip	1 serving (30g)	13	56	0.5
	Per 100g	42	185	1.8

FOOD	SERVING	CARBS (g)	CALS (kcal)	FAT (g)
Tomato Ketchup dip	1 serving (30g)	7	29	0
	Per 100g	23	96	0.1

Desserts

FOOD	SERVING	CARBS (g)	CALS (kcal)	FAT (g)
Burstin Blueberry Muffin	1 serving (120g)	49	264	5
	Per 100g	41	220	3.9
Chocolate & Vanilla Ice-Cream Sundae	1 serving (58g)	15	125	6
	Per 100g	26	216	11
Chocolate Muffin with Chocolate Chips	1 serving (120g)	48	473	28
	Per 100g	40	394	23
Crunchy Caramel Hoopla	1 serving (65g)	27	257	15
	Per 100g	42	396	23
Crunchy Chocolate Hoopla	1 serving (65g)	26	256	14
	Per 100g	40	394	21
Strawberry & Vanilla Ice-Cream Sundae	1 serving (58g)	15	119	6
	Per 100g	26	206	10
Viennetta	1 serving (300g)	36	402	27
	Per 100g	12	134	9

Biscuits

FOOD	SERVING	CARBS (g)	CALS (kcal)	FAT (g)
Buttermilk	1 biscuit (64g)	27	232	12
	Per 100g	42	363	19
Regular	1 biscuit (57g)	20	200	12
	Per 100g	35	351	21
Breadsticks	1 breadstick (35g)	17	110	3
	Per 100g	49	314	9

Calorie, Fat & Carbohydrate Counter

FOOD	SERVING	CARBS (g)	CALS (kcal)	FAT (g)
McDONALD'S				
Breakfast				
Bacon & Egg McMuffin	1 serving (141g)	27	345	18
	Per 100g	19	245	13
Bacon Roll with Brown Sauce	1 serving (118g)	37	289	9
	Per 100g	31	245	8
Big Breakfast	1 serving (256g)	41	591	36
	Per 100g	16	231	14
DBL Sausage & Egg McMuffin	1 serving (155g)	26	411	23
	Per 100g	17	265	15
DBL Bacon & Egg McMuffin	1 serving (226g)	25	572	36
	Per 100g	11	253	16
Hash Brown	1 serving (56g)	16	138	8
	Per 100g	28	247	14
Sausage & Egg McMuffin	1 serving (176g)	26	426	25
	Per 100g	15	242	14
Muffin, buttered	1 serving (63g)	26	158	4
	Per 100g	41	250	6
Muffin, buttered with preserve	1 serving (93g)	45	234	4
	Per 100g	48	252	4
Pancakes & Sausage	1 serving (262g)	89	671	26
	Per 100g	34	256	10
Meals				
Bacon McDouble with cheese	1 serving (181g)	36	478	24
	Per 100g	20	264	13
Big Mac	1 serving (215g)	45	492	23
	Per 100g	21	229	11
Cheeseburger	1 serving (122g)	33	300	12
	Per 100g	27	246	10
Chicken & Ketchup burger	1 serving (113g)	37	263	7
	Per 100g	33	233	6

FOOD	SERVING	CARBS (g)	CALS (kcal)	FAT (g)
Chicken McNuggets (4)	1 serving (72g)	8	168	10
	Per 100g	11	233	14
Chicken McNuggets (6)	1 serving (109g)	12	254	15
	Per 100g	11	233	14
Chicken McNuggets (9)	1 serving (163g)	18	380	22
	Per 100g	11	233	13
Chicken McNuggets (20)	1 serving (361g)	40	841	49
	Per 100g	11	233	14
Barbecue Dip	1 serving (32g)	12	55	0.4
	Per 100g	38	173	1.3
Mayo Dip	1 serving (24g)	0.7	182	20
	Per 100g	2.9	760	84
Mild Mustard Dip	1 serving (30g)	8	64	4
	Per 100g	25	212	13
Sweet Curry Dip	1 serving (32g)	13	61	0.8
	Per 100g	41	192	2.5
Sweet & Sour Dip	1 serving (32g)	14	59	0.3
	Per 100g	44	183	0.9
Tomato Ketchup Dip	1 serving (20g)	6	26	tr
	Per 100g	31	131	tr
Filet-O-Fish	1 serving (161g)	40	390	18
	Per 100g	25	242	11
Fish Fingers	1 serving (74g)	15	164	7
	Per 100g	20	221	9
French Fries, regular	1 serving (78g)	28	207	9
	Per 100g	36	265	12
French Fries, medium	1 serving (111g)	40	294	13
	Per 100g	36	265	12
French Fries, large	1 serving (155g)	56	411	18
	Per 100g	36	265	12
French Fries, supersize	1 serving (183g)	66	485	21
	Per 100g	36	265	11
Hamburger	1 serving (108g)	33	254	8
	Per 100g	31	235	7

Calorie, Fat & Carbohydrate Counter

FOOD	SERVING	CARBS (g)	CALS (kcal)	FAT (g)
McChicken Sandwich	1 serving (167g)	38	376	17
	Per 100g	23	225	10
Quarter Pounder with Cheese	1 serving (206g)	37	515	27
	Per 100g	18	250	13
Vegetable Deluxe	1 serving (210g)	55	422	19
	Per 100g	26	201	9

Desserts

FOOD	SERVING	CARBS (g)	CALS (kcal)	FAT (g)
Apple Pie	1 serving (80g)	26	231	13
	Per 100g	33	289	16
Birthday Cake	1 serving (64g)	45	251	7
	Per 100g	70	392	11
Donut, Chocolate	1 serving (79g)	36	329	19
	Per 100g	46	417	24
Donut, Cinnamon	1 serving (72g)	31	302	18
	Per 100g	43	419	25
Donut, Sugared	1 serving (72g)	31	303	19
	Per 100g	43	421	26
Ice Cream Cone	1 serving (98g)	24	157	5
	Per 100g	24	160	5
Ice Cream Cone with Flake	1 serving (107g)	29	204	7
	Per 100g	27	191	7
McFlurry – Crunchy	1 serving (183g)	48	320	11
	Per 100g	26	175	6
McFlurry – Dairy Milk	1 serving (182g)	44	280	13
	Per 100g	24	154	7
McFlurry – Smarties	1 serving (185g)	48	327	11
	Per 100g	26	177	6
Sundae, no topping	1 serving (149g)	33	219	7
	Per 100g	22	147	5
Sundae, hot caramel	1 serving (189g)	64	357	8
	Per 100g	34	189	4
Sundae, hot fudge	1 serving (187g)	56	352	11
	Per 100g	30	188	6

FOOD	SERVING	CARBS (g)	CALS (kcal)	FAT (g)
Sundae, strawberry	1 serving (186g)	52	296	7
	Per 100g	28	159	4

Drinks

FOOD	SERVING	CARBS (g)	CALS (kcal)	FAT (g)
Coca-Cola, regular	1 serving (250ml)	28	108	0
	Per 100ml	11	43	0
Coca-Cola, medium	1 serving (400ml)	44	172	0
	Per 100ml	11	43	0
Coca-Cola, large	1 serving (525ml)	58	226	0
	Per 100ml	11	43	0
Coca-Cola, super size	1 serving (750ml)	83	323	0
	Per 100ml	11	43	0
Diet Coke, regular	1 serving (250ml)	0	1	0
	Per 100ml	0	0.4	0
Diet Coke, medium	1 serving (500ml)	0	2	0
	Per 100ml	0	0.4	0
Diet Coke, large	1 serving (500ml)	0	2	0
	Per 100ml	0	0.4	0
Diet Coke, super size	1 serving (750ml)	0	3	0
	Per 100ml	0	0.4	0
Fanta Orange, regular	1 serving (250ml)	25	108	0
	Per 100ml	10	43	0
Fanta Orange, medium	1 serving (400ml)	40	172	0
	Per 100ml	10	43	0
Fanta Orange, large	1 serving (525ml)	53	226	0
	Per 100ml	10	43	0
Fanta Orange, super size	1 serving (750ml)	75	323	0
	Per 100ml	10	43	0
Pure Orange juice, regular	1 serving (200ml)	20	94	0
	Per 100ml	10	47	0
Pure Orange juice, large	1 serving (300ml)	30	141	0
	Per 100ml	10	47	0
Sprite, regular	1 serving (250ml)	28	108	0
	Per 100ml	11	43	0

Calorie, Fat & Carbohydrate Counter

FOOD	SERVING	CARBS (g)	CALS (kcal)	FAT (g)
Sprite, medium	1 serving (400ml)	44	172	0
	Per 100ml	11	43	0
Sprite, large	1 serving (525ml)	58	226	0
	Per 100ml	11	43	0
Sprite, super size	1 serving (750ml)	83	323	0
	Per 100ml	11	43	0
Coffee – with UHT creamer	1 serving (15ml)	0.6	18	1.5
	Per 100ml	4	123	10
Hot Chocolate Drink	1 serving (30ml)	18	101	2.7
	Per 100ml	61	336	9
Milk	1 serving (255ml)	13	125	4
	Per 100ml	5	49	1.7
Milkshake, Banana, regular	1 serving (335ml)	67	395	10
	Per 100ml	20	118	3
Milkshake, Banana, large	1 serving (430ml)	86	507	13
	Per 100ml	20	118	3
Milkshake, Chocolate, regular	1 serving (335ml)	67	402	10
	Per 100ml	20	120	3
Milkshake, Chocolate, large	1 serving (430ml)	86	516	13
	Per 100ml	20	120	3
Milkshake, Strawberry, regular	1 serving (335ml)	67	399	10
	Per 100ml	20	119	3
Milkshake, Strawberry, large	1 serving (430ml)	86	512	13
	Per 100ml	20	119	3
Milkshake, Vanilla, regular	1 serving (335ml)	64	382	10
	Per 100ml	19	114	3
Milkshake, Vanilla, large	1 serving (430ml)	82	490	13
	Per 100ml	19	114	3
Tea with skimmed milk	1 serving (15ml)	0.8	11	0.6
	Per 100ml	5	74	4

FOOD	SERVING	CARBS (g)	CALS (kcal)	FAT (g)
PIZZA EXPRESS				
Main Courses *(6 slices per pizza)*				
Pizza Margherita	Per item	87	621	21
Pizza Napolitana	Per item	87	650	23
Pizza Mushroom	Per item	87	627	21
Pizza Neptune	Per item	87	604	16
Pizza Florentina	Per item	88	724	27
Pizza Veneziana	Per item	86	613	19
Pizza Giardiniera	Per item	91	711	26
Pizza Four Seasons	Per item	87	720	29
Pizza Capricciosa	Per item	87	755	29
Pizza Caprina	Per item	92	635	22
Pizza alle Noci	Per item	89	766	35
Pizza La Reine	Per item	87	665	23
Pizza Siciliana	Per item	89	723	27
Pizza Sloppy Giuseppe	Per item	97	783	33
Pizza American	Per item	87	753	32
Pizza American Hot	Per item	87	757	33
Pizza Quattro Formaggi	Per item	87	753	22
Pizza Cajun	Per item	91	822	21
Soho Pizza	Per item	31	690	24
King Edward	Per item	44	670	36
Lasagne Pasticciate	Per item	31	499	28
Cannelloni	Per item	50	630	38
Ham & Eggs Pizza Express	Per item	45	504	24
Salade Niçoise	Per item	65	729	37
Melanzane Parmigiana	Per item	24	645	47
Side Orders				
Garlic Bread	Per item	43	227	10
Baked Dough Balls	Per item	43	200	2
Mixed Salad	Per item	5	190	18
Mozzarella & Tomato Salad	Per item	2.7	281	21

Calorie, Fat & Carbohydrate Counter

FOOD	SERVING	CARBS (g)	CALS (kcal)	FAT (g)
Caesar Salad	Per item	6	426	35
Pollo Salad	Per item	32	557	29
Tonno e Fagioli	Per item	32	337	17
Bruschetta	Per item	43	387	18

Desserts

Chocolate Fudge Cake	Per item	57	395	17
Pear Tart	Per item	41	345	18
Cheesecake	Per item	25	346	25
Tiramisu	Per item	46	456	34
Cassata	Per item	31	192	7
Bombe, Coffee & Hazelnut	Per item	24	255	14
Bombe, Chocolate & Pistachio	Per item		248	13
Bombe, Strawberry & Marsala	Per item	31	176	6
Bombe, Chocolate & Vanilla	Per item	31	246	12
Tartuffo	Per item	33	291	16

Dessert accompaniments

Vanilla Ice Cream	Per item	14	119	7
Double cream	Per item	1	188	20
Mascarpone	Per item	1	152	15

FOOD	SERVING	CARBS (g)	CALS (kcal)	FAT (g)
PIZZA HUT *(6 slices per pizza)*				
Medium Margherita (12") The Italian	1 pizza (570g)	228	1750	63
	Per 100g	40	307	11
Margherita Medium Pan Pizza	1 pizza (505g)	157	1419	61
	Per 100g	31	281	12
Vegetarian Original Medium Pan Pizza	1 pizza (560g)	157	1350	50
	Per 100g	28	241	9
Ham & Mushroom Medium (12") The Italian	1 pizza (575g)	201	1616	63
	Per 100g	35	281	11
Hawaiian Medium Pan Pizza	1 pizza (575g)	167	1443	52
	Per 100g	29	251	9
Meat Feast Medium Pan Pizza	1 pizza (685g)	164	1945	96
	Per 100g	24	284	14
Meat Feast Medium (12") The Italian	1 pizza (645g)	194	1948	90
	Per 100g	30	302	14
Supreme Medium Pan Pizza	1 pizza (635g)	159	1746	89
	Per 100g	25	275	14
Supreme Medium (12") The Italian	1 pizza (635g)	210	1778	70
	Per 100g	33	280	11
Stuffed Crust Original Margherita	1 pizza (1000g)	290	2620	100
	Per 100g	29	262	10
The Edge The Veggie	1 pizza (955g)	239	2177	86
	Per 100g	25	228	9
The Edge The Works	1 pizza (1020g)	224	2570	133
	Per 100g	22	252	13
The Edge The Meaty	1 pizza (1025g)	236	3311	185
	Per 100g	23	323	18
Garlic Bread	1 portion (90g)	43	377	19
	Per 100g	48	419	21
Garlic Bread with cheese	1 portion (165g)	50	612	35
	Per 100g	30	371	21
Chicken Wings (6)	1 portion (180g)	3.1	472	32
	Per 100g	1.7	262	18

Calorie, Fat & Carbohydrate Counter

FOOD	SERVING	CARBS (g)	CALS (kcal)	FAT (g)
BBQ dip	1 pot (25g)	7	31	0.1
	Per 100g	29	124	0.2
Garlic & Herb dip	1 pot (25g)	1.5	70	7
	Per 100g	6	280	28
Garlic Mushrooms (12)	1 portion (110g)	22	211	11
	Per 100g	20	192	10
Jacket Skins (4)	1 portion (225g)	52	574	38
	Per 100g	23	255	17
Lasagne	1 portion (445g)	62	672	31
	Per 100g	14	151	7
Spicy Chicken Bake	1 portion (425g)	81	497	13
	Per 100g	19	117	3
Tangy Tomato Bake	1 portion (425g)	94	655	21
	Per 100g	22	154	5
Dippin' Chicken (7)	1 portion (155g)	26	332	14
	Per 100g	17	214	9
Cheesy Bites – cheddar	1 bite (15g)	4.4	48	2.9
	Per 100g	29	319	19
Cheesy Bites – tomato & cheddar	1 bite (15g)	4.1	46	2.9
	Per 100g	27	308	19
Salad bar (not portioned)	1 tub (225g)	11	293	27
	Per 100g	5	130	12
Pasta Salad	1 serving (100g)	21	167	7
	Per 100g	21	167	7
Potato Salad	1 serving (100g)	15	215	17
	Per 100g	15	215	17

Desserts

Dairy Ice Cream	1 portion (140g)	32	269	13
	Per 100g	23	192	9
Fun Factory Ice Cream	1 portion (100g)	19	171	9
	Per 100g	19	171	9

8
Alphabetical listing of most common foods

Calorie, Fat & Carbohydrate Counter

FOOD	SERVING	CARBS (g)	CALS (kcal)	FAT (g)
After Eight Mints (Nestlé)	1 mint (8g)	6	34	1
	Per 100g	72	419	13
Alfalfa sprouts, raw	1 serving (85g)	0.3	21	0.6
	Per 100g	0.4	25	0.7
All Butter Shortbread (McVitie's)	1 biscuit (14g)	4	77	4
	Per 100g	30	541	30
All-Bran (Kellogg's)	Per bowl (30g)	14	81	1.2
	Per 100g	46	270	4
Almonds	1 serving (60g)	4	378	36
	Per 100g	7	630	60
Alpen (Weetabix)	Per bowl (30g)	20	110	2.1
	Per 100g	66	365	7
Anchovies, canned in oil, drained	1 Anchovy (5g)	0	14	1
	Per 100g	0	270	20
Apple juice	1 glass (200ml)	24	94	0
	Per 100ml	12	47	0
Apple pie	1 slice (about 115g)	45	302	13
	Per 100g	39	263	11
Apples, cooking stewed with sugar	1 serving (120g)	23	90	0.1
	Per 100g	19	75	0.1
Apples, cooking stewed without sugar	1 serving (120g)	10	38	0.1
	Per 100g	8	32	0.1
Apples, eating, raw, unpeeled	1 average (120g)	7	31	0.1
	Per 100g	6	26	0.1
Apricots	3 raw average (110g)	8	35	0.1
	Per 100g	7	32	0.1
Apricots, dried	3 whole average (50g)	19	80	0.3
	Per 100g	37	160	0.6
Artichoke, Jerusalem, boiled	1 medium (100g)	10	40	0
	Per 100g	10	40	0
Artichoke, globe, cooked, drained	1 medium (220g)	3.1	18	0
	Per 100g	1.4	8	0
Asparagus, fresh, boiled	5 spears (150g)	1.2	20	0
	Per 100g	0.8	13	0
Aubergine, fried in corn oil	1 serving (120g)	3.5	378	38
	Per 100g	2.9	315	32

FOOD	SERVING	CARBS (g)	CALS (kcal)	FAT (g)
Avocado pear	1 medium (145g)	2.9	290	28
	Per 100g	2	200	19
Avocado, average	1 average medium (120g)	1.6	162	17
	Per 100g	1.3	135	14
Bacon rasher, fried, middle	1 serving (160g)	0	760	72
	Per 100g	0	475	45
Bacon rasher, streaky	1 serving (160g)	0	688	64
	Per 100g	0	430	40
Bagel, egg	1 (about 60g)	33	172	1.5
	Per 100g	55	280	2.4
Baked beans, canned in tomato sauce	1 serving (85g)	13	68	0.5
	Per 100g	15	80	0.6
Baking powder	1 tbsp (25g)	9	43	0
	Per 100g	37	170	0
Banana cream pie, homemade	1 slice (about 115g)	40	285	12
	Per 100g	35	248	10
Bananas	1 average raw, peeled (140g)	32	133	0.4
	Per 100g	23	95	0.3
Basil and parmesan pasta salad	1 pack (200g)	40	260	7
	Per 100g	20	130	3.6
Basil, dried, ground	1 tsp (2g)	0.86	5.02	0.08
	Per 100g	43	251	4
Basil, fresh	1 tbsp (5g)	0.255	2	0.04
	Per 100g	5.1	40	0.8
Basmati rice, cooked	1 serving (110g)	49.5	200.2	0.44
	Per 100g	45	182	0.4
Bass, sea, mixed species	1 serving (130g)	0	150	3.3
	Per 100g	0	115	2.5
Beef liver, braised	1 serving (80g)	3	124	4
	Per 100g	3.6	155	5
Beef mince, stewed	1 serving (160g)	0	384	24
	Per 100g	0	240	15
Beef rib eye steak, lean only, broiled	1 serving (160g)	0	360	19
	Per 100g	0	225	12
Beef rump steak, fried	1 serving (160g)	0	400	24
	Per 100g	0	250	15

Calorie, Fat & Carbohydrate Counter

FOOD	SERVING	CARBS (g)	CALS (kcal)	FAT (g)
Beef sirloin, roast	1 serving (160g)	0	480	34
	Per 100g	0	300	21
Beer, average	1 pint (574ml)	13	182	0
	Per 100ml	2.3	32	0
Beer, bitter, canned	1 can 440ml	10	143	0
	Per 100ml	2.3	33	0
Beer, draught	1 pint (574ml)	13	184	0
	Per 100ml	2.3	32	0
Beetroot, raw	1 medium (120g)	8	42	0.1
	Per 100g	7	35	0.1
Black kidney beans, cooked	1 serving (85g)	20	106	0.4
	Per 100g	24	125	0.5
Black-eyed beans, cooked	1 serving (85g)	18	98	0.6
	Per 100g	21	115	0.7
Blackberries, raw	1 serving (60g)	3	16	0.1
	Per 100g	5	26	0.2
Blackberry pie	1 slice (about 115g)	41	287	13
	Per 100g	36	250	11
Blackcurrant juice, Ribena	1 carton (288ml)	40	164	0
	Per 100ml	14	57	0
Blackcurrants, raw	1 serving (60g)	4	16	tr
	Per 100g	7	27	tr
Blue Riband (Nestlé)	1 biscuit (21g)	14	109	6
	Per 100g	64	516	27
Blueberry pie	1 slice (about 115g)	41	286	13
	Per 100g	36	249	11
Boasters (McVitie's)	1 biscuit (19g)	11	104	6
	Per 100g	55	547	33
Bolognaise	1 serving (125g)	3.4	188	14
	Per 100g	2.7	150	11
Boost (Cadbury's)	1 bar (55g)	34	297	16
	Per 100g	62	540	29
Bounty (Mars)	1 bar (58g)	32	275	15
	Per 100g	56	474	26
Bovril	1 tbsp (25g)	0.7	40	0.2
	Per 100g	2.8	160	0.7

FOOD	SERVING	CARBS (g)	CALS (kcal)	FAT (g)
Bran Flakes (Kellogg's)	Per bowl (30g)	20	96	0.9
	Per 100g	66	320	3
Brazil nuts	1 serving (85g)	2.7	599	55
	Per 100g	3.2	705	65
Bread & butter pudding	1 slice (about 115g)	21	184	9
	Per 100g	18	160	8
Brie	1 portion (85g)	0.3	259	21
	Per 100g	0.3	305	25
Broad beans, fresh, cooked	1 serving (85g)	5	43	0.7
	Per 100g	6	50	0.8
Broad beans, raw	1 serving (85g)	6	51	0.9
	Per 100g	7	60	1
Broccoli, boiled in salted water	1 serving (80g)	0.9	19	0.6
	Per 100g	1.1	24	0.8
Brown bread	1 medium slice (about 30g)	13	65	0.6
	Per 100g	45	210	2
Brown bread, toasted	1 medium slice (about 30g)	17	25	0.6
	Per 100g	55	85	1.9
Brown rice, boiled	1 serving (110g)	1.2	35	2.9
	Per 100g	32	110	1.2
Brown Roll, crusty	1 (about 45g)	24	122	1.3
	Per 100g	55	275	2.9
Brown roll, soft	1 (about 45g)	25	129	1.8
	Per 100g	55	295	4
Brussels sprouts, boiled in salted water	1 serving (80g)	2.9	28	1.1
	Per 100g	3.6	35	1.4
Butter	1 serving (50g)	0	375	40
	Per 100g	0	750	80
Butter beans, boiled	1 serving (85g)	15	94	0.5
	Per 100g	18	110	0.6
Cabbage, boiled	1 serving (80g)	1.8	13	0.3
	Per 100g	2.3	16	0.4
Cabbage, Chinese, pak-choi, raw	1 serving (60g)	0	8	0
	Per 100g	0	13	0
Cabbage, red, boiled	1 serving (80g)	1.8	11	0.2
	Per 100g	2.3	14	0.3

Calorie, Fat & Carbohydrate Counter

FOOD	SERVING	CARBS (g)	CALS (kcal)	FAT (g)
Cabbage, savoy, cooked	1 serving (60g)	1	10	0.1
	Per 100g	1.7	17	0.2
Camembert	1 portion (85g)	0.3	230	20
	Per 100g	0.3	270	24
Caramel (Cadbury's)	1 bar (50g)	31	240	12
	Per 100g	61	480	24
Carrot cake	average slice (50g)	22	201	12
	Per 100g	44	402	23
Carrots, raw	1 medium (120g)	7	29	0.2
	Per 100g	6	24	0.2
Carrots, whole, boiled	1 serving (85g)	5	25	0.1
	Per 100g	6	29	0.1
Cashew nuts, dry roasted, salted	1 serving (70g)	22	396	32
	Per 100g	32	565	45
Cashew nuts, dry roasted, unsalted	1 serving (70g)	23	417	32
	Per 100g	33	595	45
Cashew nuts, oil roastd, salted	1 serving (70g)	20	406	35
	Per 100g	28	580	50
Cashew nuts, oil roasted, unsalted	1 serving (70g)	21	413	35
	Per 100g	30	590	50
Cauliflower, boiled	1 serving (80g)	1.7	22	0.7
	Per 100g	2.1	27	0.9
Cauliflower, raw	1 serving (80g)	2.4	26	0.7
	Per 100g	3	33	0.9
Caesar salad	1 pack (295g)	20	466	39
	Per 100g	7	158	13
Celeriac, boiled	1 serving (80g)	1.5	12	0.4
	Per 100g	1.9	15	0.5
Celery, raw	1 med stalk (40g)	0.4	2.8	0.1
	Per 100g	1	7	0.2
Champagne	1 small glass (125ml)	1.7	95	0
	Per 100ml	1.4	76	0
Chapatis, made with fat	1 (about 100g)	48	328	13
	Per 100g	45	315	12
Chapatis, made without fat	1 (about 100g)	44	202	1
	Per 100g	45	210	1

FOOD	SERVING	CARBS (g)	CALS (kcal)	FAT (g)
Cheddar	1 portion (85g)	1.1	327	26
	Per 100g	1.3	385	30
Cheddar, low fat	1 portion (85g)	0	264	20
	Per 100g	0	310	24
Cheddars (McVitie's)	1 biscuit (4g)	2.2	22	1.3
	Per 100g	50	540	31
Cheerios (Nestlé)	Per bowl (30g)	23	111	1.2
	Per 100g	75	369	4
Cheese Melts (Carr's)	1 biscuit (4g)	2.6	21	1
	Per 100g	58	468	22
Cheese pasta salad	1 pack (200g)	29	504	39
	Per 100g	15	252	20
Cheesecake	average slice (60g)	18	193	12
	Per 100g	30	320	20
Cherries, raw	1 serving (120g)	13	60	0.1
	Per 100g	11	50	0.1
Cherry cake	average slice (50g)	31	192	8
	Per 100g	62	384	16
Chestnuts	1 serving (70g)	25	116	1.9
	Per 100g	36	165	2.7
Chicken Balti and rice	1 pack (370g)	62	440	13
	Per 100g	17	119	3.5
Chicken Biryani	1pack (300g)	57	477	18
	Per 100g	20	159	6
Chicken Caesar salad	1 pack (300g)	32	330	14
	Per 100g	11	110	5
Chicken curry with chips	1 pack (380g)	78	475	8
	Per 100g	20.5	125	2.2
Chicken drumsticks, broiler/fryer	1 serving (160g)	0	288	10
	Per 100g	0	180	6
Chicken Jalfrezi with basmati rice	1 pack (340g)	48	391	14
	Per 100g	14	115	4
Chicken Korma and pilau rice	1 meal (450g)	66	513	10
	Per 100g	15	114	2.2
Chicken leg, broiler/fryer	1 serving (160g)	0	328	14
	Per 100g	0	205	9

Calorie, Fat & Carbohydrate Counter

FOOD	SERVING	CARBS (g)	CALS (kcal)	FAT (g)
Chicken liver pate	Per pack (113g)	3.3	370	35
	Per 100g	2.9	327	31
Chicken Madras with pilau rice, (Eastern Classics)	1 pack (400g)	59	616	29
	Per 100g	15	154	7.2
Chicken Madras, (Tesco)	1 meal (350g)	13	326	14
	Per 100g	3.6	93	4.1
Chicken pate	Per pack (175g)	3.2	408	32
	Per 100g	1.8	233	18
Chicken thigh, broiler/fryer	1 serving (160g)	0	304	16
	Per 100g	0	190	10
Chicken Tikka Masala and basmati rice	1 pack (400g)	60	580	20
	Per 100g	15	145	5
Chicken wings, broiler/fryer	1 serving (160g)	0	320	13
	Per 100g	0	200	8
Chicken, roast, meat only	1 serving (160g)	0	224	8
	Per 100g	0	140	5
Chicken, wing quarter, roast, meat only	1 serving (160g)	0	120	4
	Per 100g	0	75	2.6
Chilli	1 serving (20g)	11	9	0
	Per 100g	55	45	0
Chilli powder	1 tsp (2g)	0	0	0.34
	Per 100g	0	0	17
Chives	fresh, 2 tbsp (40g)	0.6	8	0.2
	Per 100g	1.5	19	0.6
Chocolate Buttons (Cadbury's)	1 pack (65g)	37	341	19
	Per 100g	57	525	29
Chocolate chip biscuit	5 (about 60g)	37	247	11
	Per 100g	65	436	19
Chocolate Hob Nobs (McVitie's)	1 biscuit (16g)	10	81	3.9
	Per 100g	63	499	24
Chocolate Homewheat (McVitie's)	1 biscuit (17g)	11	87	4
	Per 100g	65	505	24
Chorizo, dried	1 link (about 60g)	1.1	273	23
	Per 100g	1.9	481	41
Christmas pudding	1 slice (about 115g)	58	335	12
	Per 100g	50	291	10

FOOD	SERVING	CARBS (g)	CALS (kcal)	FAT (g)
Cider, dry	1 pint (574ml)	15	208	0
	Per 100ml	2.6	36	0
Cider, sweet	1 pint (574ml)	24	244	0
	Per 100ml	4	43	0
Cider, vintage, strong	1 pint (574ml)	42	578	0
	Per 100ml	7	101	0
Cinnamon Grahams (Nestlé)	Per bowl (30g)	23	125	3.3
	Per 100g	76	416	11
Cinnamon, ground	1 tsp (2g)	0	0	0.06
	Per 100g	0	0	3.1
Clementines, raw	1 average (120g)	11	43	0.1
	Per 100g	9	36	0.1
Coca-cola	1 glass (200ml)	21	78	0
	Per 100ml	11	39	0
Coco Pops (Kellogg's)	Per bowl (30g)	26	114	0.9
	Per 100g	85	380	3
Cocoa powder, semi-skimmed milk	1 cup (200ml)	14	114	3.8
	Per 100ml	7	57	1.9
Cocoa powder, whole milk	1 cup (200ml)	14	152	8
	Per 100ml	7	76	4
Coconut oil	1 serving (25g)	0	226	26
	Per 100g	0	905	105
Cod fillets, poached	1 serving (130g)	0	124	1.4
	Per 100g	0	95	1.1
Cod fillets, poached, weighed with skin and bone	1 serving (130g)	0	104	1.3
	Per 100g	0	80	1
Cod liver oil	1 serving (25g)	0	218	24
	Per 100g	0	870	95
Cod, baked, fillets	1 serving (130g)	0	124	1.6
	Per 100g	0	95	1.2
Cod, grilled, steaks	1 serving (130g)	0	130	1.7
	Per 100g	0	100	1.3
Cod, in batter, fried in dripping	1 serving (130g)	10	260	13
	Per 100g	8	200	10
Cod, in batter, fried in oil	1 serving (130g)	10	267	13
	Per 100g	8	205	10

Calorie, Fat & Carbohydrate Counter

FOOD	SERVING	CARBS (g)	CALS (kcal)	FAT (g)
Coffee powder, instant	1 cup (200ml)	22	200	0
	Per 100ml	11	100	0
Coffee powder, perculator	1 cup (200ml)	0.6	4	0
	Per 100ml	0.3	2	0
Coleslaw mix	1 pack (440g)	27	136	0.9
	Per 100g	6	31	0.2
Coleslaw salad	1 pack (350g)	15	305	26
	Per 100g	4	87	7
Condensed milk, skimmed, sweetened	1 glass (200ml)	120	530	0.4
	Per 100ml	60	265	0.2
Coriander, dried	1 tsp (2g)	0.8	5.6	0.09
	Per 100g	40	280	4.5
Coriander, fresh	1 tbsp (5g)	0.105	1.25	0.03
	Per 100g	2.1	25	0.7
Corn Flakes (Kellogg's)	Per bowl (30g)	25	111	0.3
	Per 100g	83	370	1
Corn oil	1 serving (25g)	0	233	26
	Per 100g	0	930	105
Corned beef	2 slices (about 60g)	0	142	9
	Per 100g	0	250	15
Cornetto	1 serving (120g)	43	306	16
	Per 100g	36	255	13
Cottage with pineapple, low fat	1 portion (85g)	9	77	0
	Per 100g	10	90	0
Courgette, boiled in unsalted water	1 serving (60g)	1.1	11	0.2
	Per 100g	1.9	19	0.4
Courgette, fried in corn oil	1 serving (60g)	1.6	39	3
	Per 100g	2.7	65	5
Crab pate	Per pack (113g)	0.6	236	19
	Per 100g	0.5	209	17
Crab, Alaskan king, steamed	1 serving (130g)	0	124	2
	Per 100g	0	95	1.5
Crab, blue, cooked	1 serving (130g)	0	130	2.2
	Per 100g	0	100	1.7
Crab, boiled	1 serving (130g)	0	156	7
	Per 100g	0	120	5

FOOD	SERVING	CARBS (g)	CALS (kcal)	FAT (g)
Crackerbread (Ryvita)	1 biscuit (5g)	4	19	0.2
	Per 100g	79	383	3
Cream cheese	1 portion (85g)	2	268	27
	Per 100g	2.3	315	32
Cream crackers	1 biscuit (8g)	6	35	1.1
	Per 100g	70	440	15
Creamed cottage	1 portion (85g)	1.4	68	2.9
	Per 100g	1.6	80	3.4
Creme Caramel	1 serving (about 115g)	24	125	2
	Per 100g	21	109	2
Crème fraiche	Per serving (80ml)	2.8	364.8	42.4
	Per 100ml	3.5	456	53
Crisp mixed salad	1 pack (390g)	12	78	1.2
	Per 100g	3	20	0.3
Croissant	1 (about 60g)	23	216	12
	Per 100g	38	355	20
Crumpet, toasted	1 (about 45g)	20	90	0.5
	Per 100g	45	195	1
Crunchie (Cadbury's)	1 bar (41g)	30	193	7
	Per 100g	72	470	18
Crunchy Nut Cornflakes (Kellogg's)	Per bowl (30g)	25	117	1.2
	Per 100g	83	390	4
Cucumber	5 average slices (80g)	1.2	8	0.1
	Per 100g	1.5	10	0.1
Curly Wurly (Cadbury's)	1 bar (29g)	20	131	5
	Per 100g	70	450	17
Currant Bread	1 slice (about 25g)	13	72	2
	Per 100g	50	290	8
Currants	1 serving (70g)	49	193	0.3
	Per 100g	70	275	0.4
Curry powder	1 tsp (2g)	0.52	4.8	0.22
	Per 100g	26	240	11
Custard Creams (Crawford's)	1 biscuit (11g)	1	7	0.4
	Per 100g	8	62	3
Custard tarts	1 tart (94g)	31	260	14
	Per 100g	33	277	15

Calorie, Fat & Carbohydrate Counter

FOOD	SERVING	CARBS (g)	CALS (kcal)	FAT (g)
Dairy Milk Chocolate (Cadbury's)	1 bar (49g)	28	260	15
	Per 100g	57	530	30
Danish pastries	1 pastry (110g)	57	411	20
	Per 100g	51	374	18
Dates, dried with stones	6 average (60g)	33	132	0.1
	Per 100g	55	220	0.2
Dessert wine – dry	1 shot glass (30ml)	1	38	0
	Per 100ml	3.3	127	0
Dessert wine – sweet	1 shot glass (30ml)	4	46	0
	Per 100ml	13	153	0
Diet Coke	1 can (330ml)	0	1	0
	Per 100ml	0	0.3	0
Diet Fanta	1 can (330ml)	0.5	5	0
	Per 100ml	0.2	1.5	0
Diet Lemonade (Schweppes)	1 bottle (500ml)	0.2	8	0
	Per 100ml	0	1.6	0
Digestive (McVitie's)	1 biscuit (15g)	10	73	3.2
	Per 100g	68	495	22
Digestive Creams (McVitie's)	1 biscuit (12g)	8	63	2.9
	Per 100g	68	507	23
Double Decker (Cadbury's)	1 bar (65g)	42	302	14
	Per 100g	65	465	21
Doughnuts, jam	1 Doughnut (75g)	37	252	11
	Per 100g	49	336	15
Doughnuts, ring	1 Doughnut (60g)	28	238	13
	Per 100g	47	397	22
Drifter (Nestlé)	1 bar (61g)	40	296	13
	Per 100g	66	486	22
Drinking chocolate, semi-skimmed milk	1 cup (200ml)	22	142	3.8
	Per 100ml	11	71	1.9
Drinking chocolate, whole milk	1 cup (200ml)	21	180	8
	Per 100ml	11	90	4
Dry Ginger Ale (Schweppes)	1 can (330ml)	13	52	0
	Per 100ml	3.9	16	0
Duck pate	Per pack (175g)	16	488	39
	Per 100g	9	279	22

FOOD	SERVING	CARBS (g)	CALS (kcal)	FAT (g)
Duck, roast, meat only	1 serving (160g)	0	312	16
	Per 100g	0	195	10
Edam	1 portion (85g)	1.1	268	23
	Per 100g	1.3	315	27
Egg fried rice	1 serving (100g)	25	210	11
	Per 100g	25	210	11
Egg, chicken, boiled	1 serving (25g)	0	36	2.8
	Per 100g	0	145	11
Egg, chicken, fried in vegetable oil	1 serving (55g)	0	96	7
	Per 100g	0	175	13
English ham	Per slice (12g)	tr	12	0.3
	Per 100g	0.3	97	2.5
English honey roast ham	Per slice (12g)	tr	18	0.8
	Per 100g	0.5	145	6
English muffin	1 (about 60g)	32	163	2.5
	Per 100g	55	265	3.9
English smoked ham	Per slice (13g)	tr	18	0.8
	Per 100g	tr	140	6
Fennel, raw	1 bulb (150g)	2.7	18	0.3
	Per 100g	1.8	12	0.2
Feta	1 portion (85g)	3.4	208	16
	Per 100g	4	245	19
Fig bars	4 (about 60g)	42	200	3.1
	Per 100g	74	353	5
Fig Rolls (Crawford's)	1 biscuit (15g)	11	60	1.6
	Per 100g	72	403	11
Figs, dried	5 average (80g)	44	180	1.3
	Per 100g	55	225	1.6
Fish cakes, fried	1 fish cake (50g)	8	90	6
	Per 100g	16	180	11
Fish fingers, fried in blended oil	1 fish finger (28g)	5	67	3.6
	Per 100g	17	240	13
Five Alive, Blackcurrant	1 carton (288ml)	44	180	0
	Per 100ml	15	63	0
Five Alive, Citrus	2 carton (288ml)	35	145	0
	Per 100ml	12	50	0

Calorie, Fat & Carbohydrate Counter

FOOD	SERVING	CARBS (g)	CALS (kcal)	FAT (g)
Five Alive, Orange Breakfast	3 carton (288ml)	31	133	0
	Per 100ml	11	46	0
Five Alive, Tropical	4 carton (288ml)	30	190	0
	Per 100ml	10	66	0
Five Alive, Very Berry	5 carton (288ml)	38	157	0
	Per 100ml	13	55	0
Flake (Cadbury's)	1 bar (34g)	19	180	11
	Per 100g	56	530	31
Four leaf salad	1 pack (140g)	2.2	20	0.6
	Per 100g	1.6	14	0.4
Frankfurter, beef	1 (about 45g)	0.8	142	13
	Per 100g	1.9	334	30
Frankfurter, chicken	1 (about 45g)	3.1	116	9
	Per 100g	7	273	21
Frankfurter, turkey	1 (about 45g)	0.7	102	8
	Per 100g	1.6	240	19
French garlic sausage	Per slice (13g)	0.1	27	2.1
	Per 100g	0.5	214	17
French or Vienna bread	1 slice (35g)	19	96	0.8
	Per 100g	55	275	2.3
French salami	Per slice (5g)	0.1	22	1.8
	Per 100g	1.9	440	36
Fresh cream, clotted	Per serving (80ml)	1.92	460	52
	Per 100ml	2.4	575	65
Fresh cream, double	Per serving (80ml)	2.16	372	36
	Per 100ml	2.7	465	45
Fresh cream, half, pasteurised	Per serving (80ml)	3.2	120	10.4
	Per 100ml	4	150	13
Fresh cream, single	Per serving (80ml)	3.04	156	15.2
	Per 100ml	3.8	195	19
Fresh cream, soured	Per serving (80ml)	3.04	156	16
	Per 100ml	3.8	195	20
Fresh cream, whipping	Per serving (80ml)	2.4	296	32
	Per 100ml	3	370	40
Frosties (Kellogg's)	Per bowl (30g)	26	111	0.3
	Per 100g	87	370	1

FOOD	SERVING	CARBS (g)	CALS (kcal)	FAT (g)
Fruit 'n' Fibre (Kellogg's)	Per bowl (30g)	21	105	1.5
	Per 100g	71	350	5
Fruit cake, iced	average slice (70g)	44	249	8
	Per 100g	62	349	11
Fruit cake, plain	average slice (70g)	40	230	8
	Per 100g	57	330	12
Fruit cake, retail	average slice (70g)	39	225	7
	Per 100g	55	315	10
Fruit cake, rich	average slice (70g)	43	239	8
	Per 100g	60	335	11
Fruit Pastilles (Rowntree)	12 sweets (53g)	44	184	0
	Per 100g	83	348	0
Fruit trifle	1 trifle (50g)	10	83	5
	Per 100g	19	166	9
Fudge (Cadbury's)	1 bar (26g)	19	116	4
	Per 100g	72	445	16
Fudge, chocolate, chocolate-coated	30g	21	120	5
	Per 100g	72	423	16
Fudge, vanilla	30g	21	111	3.1
	Per 100g	74	392	11
Galaxy Caramel (Mars)	1 bar (48g)	29	233	12
	Per 100g	60	485	25
Garden salad	1 pack (225g)	5	34	0.7
	Per 100g	2	15	0.3
Garlic, raw	2 peeled cloves (6g)	1	6	0
	Per 100g	16	95	0.6
Gateau	average slice (85g)	37	290	145
	Per 100g	44	348	174
Gelatin	1 tbsp (25g)	0	84	0
	Per 100g	0	335	0
German Salami	Per slice (8g)	tr	28	2.2
	Per 100g	0.5	331	27
Gherkins, pickled and drained	1 serving (60g)	1.6	8	0.1
	Per 100g	2.7	14	0.1
Ginger root, crystallized, candied	30g	24	95	0.1
	Per 100g	86	335	0.4

Calorie, Fat & Carbohydrate Counter

FOOD	SERVING	CARBS (g)	CALS (kcal)	FAT (g)
Goat's cheese	1 portion (85g)	1.4	162	14
	Per 100g	1.6	190	17
Golden Wonder, Wheat Crunchies, cheese	1 packet (25g)	14	138	8
	Per 100g	57	550	34
Goose, roast, meat, only	1 serving (160g)	0	520	35
	Per 100g	0	325	22
Gooseberries, raw	1 serving (120g)	3.7	22	0.5
	Per 100g	3.1	18	0.4
Granary bread	1 slice (about 25g)	12	59	0.7
	Per 100g	45	225	2.6
Grape juice, unsweetened	1 glass (200ml)	23	92	0
	Per 100ml	12	46	0
Grapefruit juice	1 glass (200ml)	17	66	0
	Per 100ml	9	33	0
Grapefruit juice, unsweetened	1 glass (200ml)	17	66	0
	Per 100ml	8	33	0
Grapefruit, raw, peeled	1/2 grapefruit (130g)	9	38	0.1
	Per 100g	7	29	0.1
Grapes	1 serving (120g)	18	72	0.1
	Per 100g	15	60	0.1
Gravy, powder	1 serving (125g)	2.6	14	0
	Per 100g	2.1	11	0
Green beans, fresh, cooked	1 serving (85g)	2.5	18	0
	Per 100g	2.9	21	0
Green beans, frozen, cooked	1 serving (85g)	4	20	0
	Per 100g	5	24	0
Green crisp salad	1 pack (180g)	3.1	29	0.9
	Per 100g	1.7	16	0.5
Gruyere	1 portion (85g)	0.3	336	25
	Per 100g	0.3	395	29
Guava, raw	1 serving (120g)	6	32	0.6
	Per 100g	5	27	0.5
Gumdrops	30g	25	100	tr
	Per 100g	88	353	tr
Haddock, in crumbs, fried in oil	1 serving (130g)	5	234	10
	Per 100g	3.7	180	8

FOOD	SERVING	CARBS (g)	CALS (kcal)	FAT (g)
Haddock, smoked, steamed	1 serving (130g)	0	130	1.2
	Per 100g	0	100	0.9
Halibut, steamed	1 serving (130g)	0	163	5
	Per 100g	0	125	4
Halloumi	1 portion (85g)	0	200	14
	Per 100g	0	235	17
Ham, cured, boneless roasted	1 serving (160g)	0.8	264	13
	Per 100g	0.5	165	8
Hamburger roll	1 (about 85g)	42	223	4
	Per 100g	50	275	5
Haricot beans, cooked	1 serving (85g)	14	77	0.4
	Per 100g	17	90	0.5
Hazelnuts	1 serving (70g)	4	434	46
	Per 100g	6	620	65
Herb salad	1 pack (100g)	1.8	16	0.5
	Per 100g	1.8	16	0.5
Hob Nobs, orginal (McVitie's)	1 biscuit (14g)	9	69	3.1
	Per 100g	64	484	22
Horlicks powder, semi-skimmed milk	1 cup (200ml)	26	162	3.8
	Per 100ml	13	81	1.9
Horlicks powder, whole milk	1 cup (200ml)	25	198	8
	Per 100ml	13	99	3.9
Hot cross buns	1 bun (about 50g)	30	155	3.4
	Per 100g	55	310	7
Hovis cracker (Jacob's)	1 biscuit (6g)	3.7	27	1.1
	Per 100g	62	454	19
Hula hoops, original	1 packet (27g)	15	140	8
	Per 100g	55	517	31
Ice cream, flavoured	1 serving (120g)	31	222	10
	Per 100g	26	185	8
Iceburg lettuce salad	1 pack (300g)	6	39	0.9
	Per 100g	1.9	13	0.3
Italian bread	1 slice (about 30g)	18	88	4
	Per 100g	55	290	14
Italian style salad	1 pack (120g)	2	17	0.6
	Per 100g	1.7	14	0.5

Calorie, Fat & Carbohydrate Counter

FOOD	SERVING	CARBS (g)	CALS (kcal)	FAT (g)
Jacobs, Twiglets, original	1 packet (125g)	77	488	14
	Per 100g	61	390	11
Jaffa Cakes (McVitie's)	1 biscuit (13g)	9	48	1
	Per 100g	74	384	8
Jam fairy	average slice (50g)	30	210	9
	Per 100g	60	420	18
Jam sponge	average slice (50g)	34	156	1.3
	Per 100g	68	312	2.5
Jam tarts	1 slice (90g)	56	342	14
	Per 100g	62	380	15
Jardin salad	1 pack (250g)	4	35	1.3
	Per 100g	1.7	14	0.5
Jarlsberg	1 portion (85g)	0	332	25
	Per 100g	0	390	29
Jelly beans	10 (30g)	26	103	0.1
	Per 100g	92	363	0.4
Kettle chips, lightly salted	1 packet (50g)	26	233	13
	Per 100g	52	465	26
Kettle chips, sea salt and balsamic vinegar	1 packet (50g)	30	234	12
	Per 100g	61	468	24
Kettle chips, sea salt and crushed black pepper	1 packet (50g)	27	239	13
	Per 100g	53	477	26
Kidney beans, red, canned, drained, heated	1 serving (85g)	9	60	0.4
	Per 100g	11	70	0.5
Kipper, baked	1 serving (130g)	0	260	14
	Per 100g	0	200	11
Kit Kat (Nestlé)	1 bar (49g)	29	246	13
	Per 100g	60	502	26
Kiwi fruit, peeled	1 small (80g)	9	40	0.4
	Per 100g	11	50	0.5
Lager, bottled	large (500ml)	8	146	0
	Per 100ml	1.5	29	0
Lamb chops, grilled	1 serving (160g)	0	576	48
	Per 100g	0	360	30
Lamb curry with rice, (Bird's Eye)	1 pack (382g)	80	520	13
	Per 100g	21	136	3.4

FOOD	SERVING	CARBS (g)	CALS (kcal)	FAT (g)
Lamb cutlets, grilled	1 serving (160g)	0	584	51
	Per 100g	0	365	32
Lamb foreshank, lean only, roasted	1 serving (160g)	0	304	10
	Per 100g	0	190	6
Lamb liver, braised	1 serving (80g)	2	184	7
	Per 100g	2.6	230	9
Lamb samosa (Waitrose)	1 oz (28g)	5	87	6
	Per 100g	18	310	23
Lamb shank, lean only, roasted	1 serving (160g)	0	272	11
	Per 100g	0	170	7
Lamb shoulder, lean and fat, roast	1 serving (160g)	0	488	43
	Per 100g	0	305	27
Lamb sirloin, lean only, roasted	1 serving (160g)	0	312	14
	Per 100g	0	195	9
Lamb stew, lean only, broiled	1 serving (160g)	0	288	11
	Per 100g	0	180	7
Lasagna, Vegetable, average	1 oz (28g)	3.5	29	1.2
	Per 100g	12.4	102	4.4
Leaf salad	1 pack (115g)	1.7	16	0.5
	Per 100g	1.5	14	0.4
Leeks, boiled in unsalted water	1 serving (60g)	1.5	13	0.4
	Per 100g	2.5	21	0.7
Lemon sole, steamed	1 serving (130g)	0	124	1.2
	Per 100g	0	95	0.9
Lemons, whole	1 large (120g)	4	22	0.4
	Per 100g	3.3	18	0.3
Lettuce, iceberg	1 serving (40g)	0.8	5	0.1
	Per 100g	1.9	12	0.3
Lettuce, raw	1 serving (40g)	0.6	6	0.2
	Per 100g	1.6	15	0.5
Lion Bar (Nestlé)	1 bar (56g)	37	270	12
	Per 100g	66	482	22
Liqueur, cream	1 shot (30ml)	6	81	0
	Per 100ml	24	324	0
Liqueur, Drambuie	1 shot (30ml)	6	79	0
	Per 100ml	24	314	0

Calorie, Fat & Carbohydrate Counter

FOOD	SERVING	CARBS (g)	CALS (kcal)	FAT (g)
Liqueur, cherry brandy/coffee	1 shot (30ml)	8	66	0
	Per 100ml	33	262	0
Lobster, boiled	1 serving (130g)	0	163	4
	Per 100g	0	125	3.4
Lobster, steamed	1 serving (130g)	1.7	124	0.8
	Per 100g	1.3	95	0.6
Lucozade	1 glass (200ml)	36	134	0
	Per 100ml	18	67	0
Lychees, raw	1 serving (120g)	17	66	0.1
	Per 100g	14	55	0.1
Macaroni, boiled	1 serving (110g)	17.6	90.2	0.55
	Per 100g	16	82	0.5
Macaroons	2 (about 45g)	25	181	9
	Per 100g	59	426	21
Mackerel, Atlantic	1 serving (130g)	0	345	22
	Per 100g	0	265	17
Mackerel, fried	1 serving (130g)	0	254	16
	Per 100g	0	195	12
Madeira Cake	1 slice (40g)	24	157	7
	Per 100g	59	393	17
Malt loaf	1 slice (about 35g)	20	94	0.8
	Per 100g	55	255	2.4
Maltesers (Mars)	1 bar (41g)	25	199	9
	Per 100g	61	486	23
Mangoes, ripe, raw	1 whole (200g)	28	120	0.4
	Per 100g	14	60	0.2
Mangoes, with skin and stone	1 large (450g)	45	171	0.5
	Per 100g	10	38	0.1
Margarine	1 serving (50g)	0.5	375	40
	Per 100g	1	750	80
Marmite	1 tbsp (25g)	0.5	41	0.2
	Per 100g	1.8	165	0.7
Marrow, boiled in unsalted water	1 serving (85g)	1.4	8	0.2
	Per 100g	1.6	9	0.2
Mars Bar (Mars)	1 bar (59g)	41	281	11
	Per 100g	70	477	18

FOOD	SERVING	CARBS (g)	CALS (kcal)	FAT (g)
Marzipan	1 serving (50g)	25	220	13
	Per 100g	50	440	26
Mayonnaise	1 tbsp (25g)	0.4	173	19
	Per 100g	1.7	690	75
Mcvites, Mini Cheddars	1 packet (50g)	27	268	15
	Per 100g	54	535	30
Mediterranean style bean and smoked tomato salad	1 pack (225g)	28	414	29
	Per 100g	13	184	13
Mediterranean pasta salad	1 pack (350g)	34	305	16
	Per 100g	10	87	5
Melon, cantaloupe	1 serving (160g)	6	30	0.2
	Per 100g	3.9	19	0.1
Melon, galia	1 serving (160g)	10	40	0.2
	Per 100g	6	25	0.1
Melon, honeydew	1 serving (160g)	11	43	0.2
	Per 100g	7	27	0.1
Melon, watermelon	1 serving (160g)	11	48	0.5
	Per 100g	7	30	0.3
Melts (Carr's)	1 biscuit (4g)	2.3	19	0.9
	Per 100g	58	451	20
Meringue	1 serving (25g)	25	93	0
	Per 100g	100	370	0
Milk Chocolate Aero (Nestlé)	1 bar (39g)	22	202	11
	Per 100g	57	518	29
Milk Chocolate Yorkie (Nestlé)	1 bar (70g)	41	368	21
	Per 100g	59	526	30
Milk shake powder, semi-skimmed milk	1 cup (200ml)	23	138	3.2
	Per 100ml	11	69	1.6
Milk shake powder, whole milk	1 cup (200ml)	22	174	7
	Per 100ml	11	87	3.7
Milky Way (Mars)	1 bar (26g)	19	116	4
	Per 100g	72	447	16
Mince pie	1 pie (about 50g)	28	183	8
	Per 100g	56	366	15
Mince pies (Mr Kipling)	1 pie (62g)	35	231	9
	Per 100g	54	372	14

Calorie, Fat & Carbohydrate Counter

FOOD	SERVING	CARBS (g)	CALS (kcal)	FAT (g)
Mini Ritz Crackers (Jacob's)	1 biscuit (3g)	1.8	17	1
	Per 100g	56	534	32
Mint sauce	1 tbsp (25g)	5	23	0
	Per 100g	21	90	0
Mint, fresh	1 tbsp (5g)	0.25	2	0.03
	Per 100g	5	40	0.7
Mixed vegetables, frozen, boiled	1 serving (85g)	6	38	0.4
	Per 100g	7	45	0.5
Mozzarella, part-skim	1 portion (85g)	2.3	191	14
	Per 100g	2.7	225	17
Mozzarella, whole-milk	1 portion (85g)	1.7	213	17
	Per 100g	2	250	20
Mushrooms, boiled in salted water	1 serving (60g)	0.2	7	0.2
	Per 100g	0.4	11	0.3
Mushrooms, common, raw	1 serving (60g)	0.2	8	0.3
	Per 100g	0.4	13	0.5
Mushrooms, fried in corn oil	1 serving (60g)	0.2	96	10
	Per 100g	0.3	160	16
Mussels, boiled	1 serving (130g)	tr	117	2.6
	Per 100g	tr	90	2
Mustard powder	1 tsp (2g)	0.42	9.3	0.6
	Per 100g	21	465	30
Mustard, smooth	1 tbsp (25g)	2.5	34	2
	Per 100g	10	135	8
Mustard, wholegrain	1 tbsp (25g)	1	34	2.5
	Per 100g	4	135	10
Naan bread	1 (about 160g)	80	538	20
	Per 100g	50	345	13
Nectarines	1 average (120g)	11	48	0.1
	Per 100g	9	40	0.1
Noodles, egg, boiled	1 serving (110g)	13.2	77	0.55
	Per 100g	12	70	0.5
Noodles, rice, boiled	1 serving (110g)	27.5	112.2	0.55
	Per 100g	25	102	0.5
Noodles, rice, fried	1 serving (150g)	19.5	240	18
	Per 100g	13	160	12

FOOD	SERVING	CARBS (g)	CALS (kcal)	FAT (g)
Nutmeg, ground	1 tsp (2g)	0	0	0.74
	Per 100g	0	0	37
Octopus, common	1 serving (130g)	2.7	111	1.4
	Per 100g	2.1	85	1.1
Olive oil	1 serving (25g)	0	233	24
	Per 100g	0	930	95
Olives, black	5 large (20g)	1.4	24	2.4
	Per 100g	7	120	12
Olives, green, unstuffed	5 large (18g)	0.3	27	2.9
	Per 100g	1.7	150	16
Omelette, cheese	1 serving (100g)	0	255	23
	Per 100g	0	255	23
Omelette, plain	1 serving (100g)	0	185	16
	Per 100g	0	185	16
Onions, fried in blended oil	1 serving (60g)	8	102	7
	Per 100g	14	170	11
Onions, raw	1 serving (60g)	5	21	0.1
	Per 100g	8	35	0.2
Orange juice	1 glass (200ml)	18	72	0
	Per 100ml	9	36	0
Original Ryvita	1 biscuit (9g)	0.5	2.4	0
	Per 100g	6	27	0
Ovaltine powder, semi-skimmed milk	1 cup (200ml)	26	158	3.4
	Per 100ml	13	79	1.7
Ovaltine powder, whole milk	1 cup (200ml)	26	194	8
	Per 100ml	13	97	3.8
Oxo cubes	1 tbsp (25g)	3	55	0.8
	Per 100g	12	220	3.3
Oysters, raw	10 average (60g)	0.5	69	2.3
	Per 100g	0.8	115	3.9
Palm oil	1 serving (25g)	0	219	25
	Per 100g	0	875	100
Parma ham	Per slice (13g)	tr	37	2.5
	Per 100g	0.1	275	19
Parmesan, grated	1 portion (85g)	0.6	349	25
	Per 100g	0.7	410	29

Calorie, Fat & Carbohydrate Counter

FOOD	SERVING	CARBS (g)	CALS (kcal)	FAT (g)
Parsley, fresh	1 tbsp (5g)	0.135	1.65	0.06
	Per 100g	2.7	33	1.3
Parsnip, boiled in unsalted water	1 serving (85g)	10	55	1
	Per 100g	12	65	1.2
Parsnip, raw	1 average (160g)	21	104	1.8
	Per 100g	13	65	1.1
Partridge, roast, meat only	1 serving (160g)	0	328	11
	Per 100g	0	205	7
Passion fruit	1 serving (120g)	7	42	0.5
	Per 100g	6	35	0.4
Pasta arrabbiata	1 pack (205g)	25	144	2.5
	Per 100g	12	70	1.2
Pasta bake	1 pack (250g)	25	215	9
	Per 100g	9	86	3.9
Pastrami slices	Per slice (10g)	tr	12	0.3
	Per 100g	tr	124	3
Peaches, raw	1 whole (160g)	13	51	0.2
	Per 100g	8	32	0.1
Peanut butter, smooth	1 serving (50g)	7	310	28
	Per 100g	14	620	55
Peanut butter, biscuit	4 (about 50g)	28	245	14
	Per 100g	56	494	28
Peanuts, chocolate-coated	12 (about 30g)	11	157	12
	Per 100g	39	554	41
Peanuts, dry roasted	1 serving (70g)	7	406	35
	Per 100g	10	580	50
Peanuts, dry, roasted and salted	1 serving (70g)	5	410	35
	Per 100g	7	585	50
Peanuts, plain	1 serving (70g)	8	399	32
	Per 100g	12	570	45
Pears, raw	1 average (180g)	18	70	0.2
	Per 100g	10	39	0.1
Penguin biscuits (McVitie's)	1 biscuit (24g)	16	131	7
	Per 100g	65	536	29
Pepperoni	10 slices(about 60g)	1.6	273	24
	Per 100g	2.8	481	43

FOOD	SERVING	CARBS (g)	CALS (kcal)	FAT (g)
Peppers, capsicum, chilli, green, raw	1 average (20g)	0.1	4	0.1
	Per 100g	0.7	20	0.6
Pesto	1 serving (30g)	9	90	5
	Per 100g	30	300	17
Pickle, sweet	1 tbsp (25g)	9	34	0.1
	Per 100g	34	135	0.3
Pickles, dill	1 (about 60g)	2.7	12	0.1
	Per 100g	5	21	0.2
Pickles, sour	1 (about 30g)	0.8	4	0.1
	Per 100g	2.8	13	0.3
Pickles, sweet	1 (about 30g)	11	41	0.1
	Per 100g	35	140	0.3
Picnic (Cadbury's)	1 bar (48g)	28	228	12
	Per 100g	59	475	24
Pine nuts	1 serving (25g)	1	178	18
	Per 100g	3.9	710	70
Pineapple juice, unsweetened	1 glass (200ml)	21	82	0
	Per 100ml	11	41	0
Pineapple, raw, peeled	1 slice (120g)	12	48	0.2
	Per 100g	10	40	0.2
Pistachio nuts	1 serving (70g)	18	420	35
	Per 100g	25	600	50
Pita bread (white)	1 pocket (75g)	41	203	0.9
	Per 100g	55	270	1.2
Plaice, in batter, fried in blended oil	1 serving (130g)	18	351	22
	Per 100g	14	270	17
Plaice, steamed	1 serving (130g)	0	117	2.6
	Per 100g	0	90	2
Plain Chocolate Digestive Caramels (McVitie's)	1 biscuit (17g)	11	83	3.8
	Per 100g	66	481	22
Plain Chocolate Ginger Nuts (McVitie's)	1 biscuit (14g)	10	70	2.9
	Per 100g	72	489	20
Plain Chocolate Hob Nobs (McVitie's)	1 biscuit (19g)	12	96	5
	Per 100g	63	498	24
Plain Chocolate Homewheat (McVitie's)	1 biscuit (17g)	12	88	4
	Per 100g	66	507	24

Calorie, Fat & Carbohydrate Counter

FOOD	SERVING	CARBS (g)	CALS (kcal)	FAT (g)
Plums, raw	1 average (110g)	10	39	0.1
	Per 100g	9	35	0.1
Pork chops, grilled	1 serving (160g)	0	520	40
	Per 100g	0	325	25
Pork leg, roast	1 serving (160g)	0	440	34
	Per 100g	0	275	21
Pork liver, braised	1 serving (80g)	3	128	3
	Per 100g	3.7	160	4
Pork sirloin, lean only, roasted	1 serving (160g)	0	392	21
	Per 100g	0	245	13
Pork spareribs, lean only, braised	1 serving (160g)	0	632	50
	Per 100g	0	395	31
Porridge, made with milk	Per bowl (30g)	4	35	1.5
	Per 100g	14	115	5
Porridge, made with water	Per bowl (30g)	2.7	15	0.3
	Per 100g	9	50	1
Potato salad	1 pack (32g)	2	26	2
	Per 100g	8	81	5
Potato, baked, jacket	1 serving (150g)	21	113	1.1
	Per 100g	14	75	0.7
Potato, chips, oven cook	1 serving (100g)	26	130	3
	Per 100g	26	130	3
Potato, hash brown	1 serving (55g)	14	176	12
	Per 100g	26	320	22
Potato, new, peeled	1 serving (165g)	20	99	0
	Per 100g	12	60	0
Potato, roast, no skin	1 serving (150g)	27	165	4
	Per 100g	18	110	2.8
Prawns, boiled	1 serving (130g)	0	143	2.5
	Per 100g	0	110	1.9
Pringles, original	1 packet (200g)	96	1114	76
	Per 100g	48	557	38
Prunes, ready to eat	1 serving (160g)	56	232	0.6
	Per 100g	35	145	0.4
Pumpkin and squash kernels	1 serving (70g)	13	396	32
	Per 100g	18	565	45

FOOD	SERVING	CARBS (g)	CALS (kcal)	FAT (g)
Pumpkin, boiled in salted water	1 serving (85g)	1.8	12	0.3
	Per 100g	2.1	14	0.3
Quality Street (Nestlé)	1 box (125g)	84	583	26
	Per 100g	67	466	21
Radish, raw	4 average (60g)	1.1	7	0.1
	Per 100g	1.8	12	0.2
Raisin bread	1 slice (about 30g)	14	70	0.4
	Per 100g	45	240	1.4
Raisins	1 serving (70g)	49	189	0.3
	Per 100g	70	270	0.4
Raisins, chocolate-coated	30 (about 30g)	20	119	5
	Per 100g	69	420	17
Raspberries, raw	1 serving (60g)	3	16	0.2
	Per 100g	5	26	0.3
Ready Brek (Weetabix)	Per bowl (30g)	7	107	2.4
	Per 100g	24	356	8
Red pepper and coriander couscous	1 pack (200g)	54	282	3.2
	Per 100g	27	141	1.6
Revels (Mars)	1 pack (35g)	23	171	8
	Per 100g	66	489	23
Ribena, undiluted	1 serving (50ml)	30	114	0
	Per 100ml	61	228	0
Rice Krispies (Kellogg's)	Per bowl (30g)	26	111	0.3
	Per 100g	87	370	1
Rich Tea Biscuits (McVitie's)	1 biscuit (8g)	6	39	1.3
	Per 100g	76	475	16
Roast chicken salad	1 pack (300g)	21	348	22
	Per 100g	7	116	7
Rocket salad	1 pack (100g)	0.8	11	0.5
	Per 100g	0.8	11	0.5
Roll or bun, homemade	1 (about 35g)	19	118	0.9
	Per 100g	55	350	2.4
Root beer	1 can (360ml)	39	152	0
	Per 100ml	11	42	0
Roquefort	1 portion (85g)	1.7	281	25
	Per 100g	2	330	29

Calorie, Fat & Carbohydrate Counter

FOOD	SERVING	CARBS (g)	CALS (kcal)	FAT (g)
Rosemary, dried	1 tbsp (5g)	2.25	15.75	0.8
	Per 100g	45	315	16
Roses (Cadbury's)	1 box (125g)	76	619	31
	Per 100g	61	495	25
Rum, average, 40% volume	1 shot (25ml)	0	55	0
	Per 100ml	0	220	0
Runner beans, fresh, cooked	1 serving (85g)	2	14	0.4
	Per 100g	2.4	17	0.5
Rye bread	1 slice (25g)	11	55	0.5
	Per 100g	45	220	1.8
Sage, dried, ground	1 tbsp (5g)	2.25	15.75	0.65
	Per 100g	45	315	13
Salad cream	1 tbsp (25g)	4	89	8
	Per 100g	16	355	31
Salad cream, reduced calorie	1 tbsp (25g)	2.3	50	4
	Per 100g	9	200	17
Salami, beef	2 slices (about 60g)	1.6	148	12
	Per 100g	2.8	261	21
Salami, pork	3 slices (about 60g)	0.9	230	19
	Per 100g	1.6	406	34
Salami, turkey	2 slices (about 60g)	0.3	111	8
	Per 100g	0.5	196	14
Salmon, canned	1 serving (130g)	0	195	10
	Per 100g	0	150	8
Salt, block	1 tbsp (25g)	0	0	0
	Per 100g	0	0	0
Salt, table	1 tbsp (25g)	0	0	0
	Per 100g	0	0	0
Sandwiches, cheddar cheese ploughmans	1 pack (194g)	46	456	24
	Per 100g	24	235	12
Sandwiches, cheese and celery	1 pack (179g)	26.	465	31
	Per 100g	15	260	17
Sandwiches, cheese and coleslaw	1 pack (185g)	33	500	32
	Per 100g	18	270	17
Sandwiches, chicken and sweetcorn	1 pack (140g)	28	294	14
	Per 100g	20	210	10

FOOD	SERVING	CARBS (g)	CALS (kcal)	FAT (g)
Sandwiches, coronation chicken	1 pack (210g)	42	420	20
	Per 100g	20	200	10
Sandwiches, free range egg and cress	1 pack (180g)	37	270	10
	Per 100g	21	150	6
Sandwiches, free range egg and bacon	1 pack (257g)	39	655	40
	Per 100g	15	255	16
Sandwiches, tuna salad	1 pack (250g)	42	575	32
	Per 100g	17	230	13
Sandwiches, turkey and ham	1 pack (182g)	31	410	23
	Per 100g	17	225	12
Satsumas	1 average (120g)	11	44	0.1
	Per 100g	9	37	0.1
Saucisson Montague	Per slice (5g)	0.1	21	1.8
	Per 100g	1.9	421	37
Sausage, pork, fresh	4 links (about 60g)	0.5	192	16
	Per 100g	0.9	339	29
Scampi, in breadcrumbs, frozen, fried	1 serving (130g)	26	383	20
	Per 100g	20	295	15
Scottish smoked wild venison	Per slice (20g)	0.4	41	2.1
	Per 100g	2	203	10
Semi-skimmed milk, average	1 glass (200ml)	10	90	3
	Per 100ml	5	45	1.5
Semi-skimmed milk, pasteurised	1 glass (200ml)	10	100	3.2
	Per 100ml	5	50	1.6
Sesame oil	1 serving (25g)	0	216	26
	Per 100g	0	865	105
Sesame Ryvita	1 biscuit (9g)	0.5	2.8	0.1
	Per 100g	5	31	1
Sesame seeds	1 serving (40g)	0.4	250	24
	Per 100g	0.9	625	60
Shandy, canned	large (500ml)	15	55	0
	Per 100ml	3	*1	0
Shortbread	5 (about 35g)	24	187	9
	Per 100g	69	528	25
Shreddies	Per bowl (30g)	22	103	0.6
	Per 100g	72	343	2

Calorie, Fat & Carbohydrate Counter

FOOD	SERVING	CARBS (g)	CALS (kcal)	FAT (g)
Shrimp, mixed species, fried	1 serving (90g)	11	212	11
	Per 100g	12	235	12
Skimmed milk, average	1 glass (200ml)	10	64	0.2
	Per 100ml	5	32	0.1
Snickers (Mars)	1 bar (64g)	35	321	18
	Per 100g	55	502	28
Sole	1 serving (130g)	0	150	2
	Per 100g	0	115	1.5
Sorbet, lemon	1 serving (120g)	40	162	0
	Per 100g	33	135	0
Sourdough bread	1 slice (30g)	12	74	11
	Per 100g	40	245	38
Soy sauce	1 tbsp (25g)	2	16	0
	Per 100g	8	65	0
Soya milk, plain	1 glass (200ml)	1.6	64	3.8
	Per 100ml	0.8	32	1.9
Soya oil	1 serving (25g)	0	234	25
	Per 100g	0	935	100
Spaghetti and meat balls	1 pack (900g)	135	1035	36
	Per 100g	15	115	4
Spaghetti and vegetarian meatballs	1 pack (350g)	48	382	13
	Per 100g	14	109	3.8
Spaghetti Bolognaise, average	1 oz (28g)	23	96	0
	Per 100g	81	341	0.01
Spaghetti, white, boiled	1 serving (110g)	70.4	350.9	2.64
	Per 100g	64	319	2.4
Special K (Kellogg's)	Per bowl (30g)	23	111	0.3
	Per 100g	76	370	1
Spinach, frozen, boiled in unsalted water	1 serving (60g)	0.3	13	0.5
	Per 100g	0.5	21	0.8
Spirits, average, 37.5% volume	1 shot (25ml)	0	51	0
	Per 100ml	0	204	0
Sponge cake	average slice (60g)	33	275	16
	Per 100g	55	457	27
Sponge cake, fat free	average slice (60g)	32	175	4
	Per 100g	53	291	7

FOOD	SERVING	CARBS (g)	CALS (kcal)	FAT (g)
Stout, bottled	small (275ml)	11	100	0
	Per 100ml	4	36	0
Strawberries	1 serving (60g)	3.6	16	0.1
	Per 100g	6	27	0.1
Sugar Puffs (Quaker)	Per bowl (30g)	26	116	0.3
	Per 100g	85	387	1
Sultanas	1 serving (70g)	49	193	0.3
	Per 100g	70	275	0.4
Sundried tomato potato salad	1 pack (250g)	35	490	37
	Per 100g	14	196	15
Sunflower seeds	1 serving (70g)	13	392	35
	Per 100g	18	560	50
Sweet potato, boiled in salted water	1 serving (85g)	18	72	0.3
	Per 100g	21	85	0.3
Sweetcorn, on-the-cob, boiled	1 serving (60g)	7	39	0.8
	Per 100g	12	65	1.4
Swiss	1 portion (85g)	2.8	306	22
	Per 100g	3.3	360	26
Swiss roll	average slice (35g)	24	115	2.5
	Per 100g	70	334	7
Table Water Biscuits, large (Carr's)	1 biscuit (7g)	6	33	0.7
	Per 100g	77	441	9
Table Water Biscuits, small (Carr's)	1 biscuit (3g)	2.6	15	0.3
	Per 100g	77	445	9
Tangerines	1 average (120g)	7	30	0.1
	Per 100g	6	25	0.1
Taramasalata	1 serving (50g)	2	223	25
	Per 100g	3.9	445	50
Thyme, dried, ground	1 serving (5g)	2.25	14.25	0.35
	Per 100g	45	285	7
Time Out (Cadbury's)	1 finger (18g)	5	97	11
	Per 100g	29	540	62
Toffee Crisp (Nestlé)	1 bar (49g)	30	242	13
	Per 100g	62	494	26
Tomato juice	1 glass (200ml)	6	28	0
	Per 100ml	3	14	0

Calorie, Fat & Carbohydrate Counter

FOOD	SERVING	CARBS (g)	CALS (kcal)	FAT (g)
Tomato ketchup	1 tbsp (25g)	6	24	0
	P er 100g	24	95	0
Tomato puree	1 serving (60g)	8	42	0.1
	Per 100g	13	70	0.2
Tomato sauce	1 tbsp (25g)	2.3	23	1.5
	Per 100g	9	90	6
Tomatoes, canned, whole	1 serving (85g)	2.5	14	0.1
	Per 100g	2.9	16	0.1
Tomatoes, raw	1 tomato (120g)	3.7	20	0.4
	Per 100g	3.1	17	0.3
Trout, brown, steamed	1 serving (130g)	0	169	7
	Per 100g	0	130	5
Trout, rainbow, cooked dry heat	1 serving (130g)	0	195	5
	Per 100g	0	150	4
Tuna and sweetcorn	1 pack (200g)	34	230	5
	Per 100g	17	115	2.7
Tuna and sweetcorn pasta snack	1 pack (300g)	52	609	37
	Per 100g	17	203	12
Tuna pate	Per pack (113g)	0.1	387	35
	Per 100g	0.1	342	31
Tuna salad	1 pack (370g)	35	466	29
	Per 100g	9	126	8
Tuna, canned in brine, drained	1 serving (130g)	0	130	0.8
	Per 100g	0	100	0.6
Tuna, canned in oil, drained	1 serving (130g)	0	247	12
	Per 100g	0	190	9
Tuna, fresh	1 serving (130g)	0	234	8
	Per 100g	0	180	6
Turkey ham	2 slices (about 60g)	0.2	73	2.8
	Per 100g	0.4	129	5
Turkey, roast, meat only	1 serving (160g)	0	224	4
	Per 100g	0	140	2.8
Turnip, boiled in unsalted water	1 serving (85g)	1.8	11	0.2
	Per 100g	2.1	13	0.2
Twirl (Cadbury's)	1 bar (44g)	25	231	13
	Per 100g	56	525	30

FOOD	SERVING	CARBS (g)	CALS (kcal)	FAT (g)
Twix (Mars)	1 finger (29g)	19	144	7
	Per 100g	64	495	24
Vegetable oil, average	1 serving (25g)	0	226	25
	Per 100g	0	905	100
Viennetta Chocolate (Wall's)	1 serving (55g)	13	138	8
	Per 100g	24	250	15
Vinegar	1 tbsp (25g)	0.2	1	0
	Per 100g	0.6	3.9	0
Vodka, average, 40% volume	1 shot (25ml)	0	55	0
	Per 100ml	0	220	0
Wafer thin honey roast ham	Per slice (10g)	0.2	44	0.3
	Per 100g	1.5	440	2.6
Wafer thin honey roast turkey	Per slice (10g)	0.3	55	0.4
	Per 100g	3	550	4
Wafer thin honey smoked ham	Per slice (10g)	tr	41	0.2
	Per 100g	0.5	414	2.4
Wafer thin roast chicken	Per slice (10g)	0.3	55	0.5
	Per 100g	3	552	5
Wafer thin smoked turkey	Per slice (10g)	0.2	53	0.4
	Per 100g	1.6	527	4
Waldorf salad	1 pack (250g)	23	455	38
	Per 100g	9	182	15
Walkers, Quavers	1 packet (20g)	12	103	6
	Per 100g	61	515	29
Walkers, cheese and onion	1 packet (34g)	17	179	11
	Per 100g	50	525	33
Walkers, Monster Munch, ready salted	1 packet (28g)	6	132	6
	Per 100g	22	470	22
Walkers, prawn skips	1 packet (19g)	11	98	6
	Per 100g	60	517	29
Walkers, ready salted	1 packet (35g)	17	186	12
	Per 100g	49	530	34
Walkers, roast chicken	1 packet (34g)	17	179	11
	Per 100g	50	525	33
Walkers, salt and vinegar	1 packet (34g)	17	179	11
	Per 100g	50	525	33

Calorie, Fat & Carbohydrate Counter

FOOD	SERVING	CARBS (g)	CALS (kcal)	FAT (g)
Walkers, smokey bacon	1 packet (34g)	17	179	11
	Per 100g	50	525	33
Walnuts	1 serving (70g)	2.3	462	49
	Per 100g	3.3	660	70
Watercress, raw	1 serving (60g)	0.2	14	0.6
	Per 100g	0.4	23	1
Watercress, spinach and rocket	1 pack (135g)	1.1	30	1.1
	Per 100g	0.8	22	0.8
Weetabix (Weetabix)	Per bowl (30g)	20	102	0.9
	Per 100g	68	340	3
Wensleydale	1 portion (85g)	0	310	26
	Per 100g	0	365	31
Wheatgerm loaf	1 slice (25g)	11	59	0.8
	Per 100g	45	235	3.3
Wheatgerm oil	1 serving (25g)	0	235	25
	Per 100g	0	940	100
Whisky, average, 40% volume	1 shot (25ml)	0	55	0
	Per 100ml	0	220	0
White bread, average	1 slice (30g)	15	74	0.6
	Per 100g	50	245	1.9
White bread, french stick	2" stick (40g)	22	110	1.1
	Per 100g	55	275	2.8
White rice, easy cook, boiled	1 serving (110g)	1.4	34	2.9
	Per 100g	29	133	1.2
White roll, crusty	1 (50g)	30	133	1.1
	Per 100g	60	265	2.2
White roll, soft	1 (50g)	28	135	1.9
	Per 100g	55	270	3.7
Whitebait, fried	1 serving (130g)	7	696	65
	Per 100g	5	535	50
Whitefish, mixed species, cooked in dry heat	1 serving (130g)	0	137	1.2
	Per 100g	0	105	0.9
Whole milk, average	1 glass (200ml)	10	130	8
	Per 100ml	5	65	3.9
Wholemeal bread	1 slice (25g)	10	53	0.6
	Per 100g	40	210	2.4

FOOD	SERVING	CARBS (g)	CALS (kcal)	FAT (g)
Wholemeal roll	1 (50g)	23	120	1.6
	Per 100g	45	240	3.1
Wild rocket	1 pack (50g)	0.3	9	0.2
	Per 100g	0.6	18	0.3
Wine, fortified, port	1 shot glass (50ml)	6	80	0
	Per 100ml	12	160	0
Wine, fortified, sherry, dry	1 shot glass (50ml)	0.7	58	0
	Per 100ml	1.4	116	0
Wine, fortified, sherry, medium	1 shot glass (50ml)	3	60	0
	Per 100ml	6	120	0
Wine, fortified, sherry, sweet	1 shot glass (50ml)	3.5	68	0
	Per 100ml	7	136	0
Wine, red	1 small glass (120ml)	0.4	85	0
	Per 100ml	0.3	71	0
Wine, rose	1 small glass (120ml)	3.1	89	0
	Per 100ml	2.6	74	0
Wine, white, dry	1 small glass (120ml)	0.7	82	0
	Per 100ml	0.6	68	0
Wine, white, medium	1 small glass (120ml)	4	94	0
	Per 100ml	3.6	78	0
Wine, white, sweet	1 small glass (120ml)	7	118	0
	Per 100ml	6	98	0
Wispa (Cadbury's)	1 bar (39g)	21	215	13
	Per 100g	54	550	34
Wotsits, cheesy flavour	1 packet (21g)	11	114	7
	Per 100g	51	541	34
Yeast, dried	1 tbsp (25g)	0.9	41	0.4
	Per 100g	3.7	165	1.4
Yogurt, bio type, low fat, honey	1 serving (100g)	13	100	3
	Per 100g	13	100	3
Yogurt, black cherry, with live cultures	1 serving (100g)	17	104	4
	Per 100g	17	104	4
Yogurt, drinking	1 serving (100g)	13	81	1
	Per 100g	13	81	1
Yogurt, frozen, fruit	1 serving (250g)	20	132	5
	Per 100g	8	53	2